SpringerBriefs in Molecular Science

Chemistry of Foods

Series editor

Salvatore Parisi, Palermo, Italy

More information about this series at http://www.springer.com/series/11853

Giampiero Barbieri · Caterina Barone
Arpan Bhagat · Giorgia Caruso
Zachary Ryan Conley · Salvatore Parisi

The Influence of Chemistry on New Foods and Traditional Products

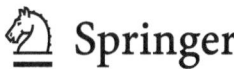 Springer

Giampiero Barbieri
Experimental Station for the Food
    Preserving Industry
Parma
Italy

Caterina Barone
ENFAP Comitato Regionale Sicilia
Palermo
Italy

Arpan Bhagat
Butterfield Foods
Indianapolis, IN
USA

Giorgia Caruso
Palermo
Italy

Zachary Ryan Conley
Stowers Institute for Medical Research
Kansas City, MO
USA

Salvatore Parisi
Gambino Industrie Alimentari S.p.A
Palermo
Italy

ISSN 2199-689X   ISSN 2199-7209   (electronic)
ISBN 978-3-319-11357-9   ISBN 978-3-319-11358-6   (eBook)
DOI 10.1007/978-3-319-11358-6

Library of Congress Control Number: 2014949362

Springer Cham Heidelberg New York Dordrecht London

Springer is part of Springer Science+Business Media (www.springer.com)

Contents

Chapter 1
The Problem of Aqueous Absorption in Processed Cheeses: A Simulated Approach

Abstract The production of fresh cheeses has always been in relation to the problem of the determination of cheesemaking yields in terms of kilograms of product per 100 l of original milk. Studies have been carried out in the past in regard to stretched cheeses using cow milk. However, there is little literature on the production and related yields of so-called 'analogue' or 'processed' cheeses. This argument can be interesting from the viewpoint of the cheesemaking industry. On the other hand, the increasing perplexity of the normal consumer should be considered because of the possibility of purchasing analogue cheeses. These products are surely a declared imitation of traditional cheeses, but they often appear as 'ameliorated' versions of the original food. From the analytical viewpoint, the maximum predictable aqueous absorption for milk proteins, especially caseins, seems one of the key points. Consequently, a simulated study on processed cheeses and separated ingredients—rennet caseins above all—can be carried out with the aim of explaining several of the unknown features of analogue cheeses.

Keywords Analogue cheese · Apparent hydric absorption · Casein · Cheesemaking yield · Hydrolysis · Moisture

Abbreviations

A%	Apparent hydric absorption
Ca^{2+}	Calcium
$CaCl_2$	Calcium chloride
CY	Cheesemaking yield
CYPEP:2006	Cheesemaking yield and proteins estimation according to Parisi: 2006

© The Author(s) 2014
G. Barbieri et al., *The Influence of Chemistry on New Foods and Traditional Products*, Chemistry of Foods, DOI 10.1007/978-3-319-11358-6_1

CCS	Compact cheese spreadsheets
DM	Dry matter
FDM	Fat content on dry matter
GSFS	Global standard for food safety
IDF	International dairy federation
IFS	International featured standards
MC	Moisture content
MFFB	Moisture on free fat basis
MW	Molecular weight
MRA	Most reliable amount
TP_{MRA}	Most reliable amount of proteins
CAS_{HA}	Presumptive 'high-adsorption' casein
$p\text{-}CAS_{HA}$	Presumptive 'high-absorption' pre-casein
RGT	Rennet gelation time
R&C	Rigorous and corrected

1.1 The Production of Cheeses: Differences Between Artisanal Products and Industrial Foods

At present, the market of cheeses and dairy products seems exposed to cyclic periods with the notable diminution of stored raw materials and the related growth of prices for finished products. In recent years, the continuity of these periods has been repeatedly interrupted during time with the consequent overproduction of cheeses and other dairy foods. The above-mentioned situation depends on the current economic crisis on a worldwide scale, but other concomitant causes have surely their weight. With reference to milk products, the cyclic deficiency of cow's milk in several countries determines the subsequent exiguity of correlated derivatives (butters, caseins, yoghurts, cheeses, etc.), but other factors should be taken into account.

With exclusive reference to dairy products—animal butters, casein products, lactose and so on—cow milk is surely the most used raw material, but other milk can be produced on a large scale with different uses [1]:

- Goat milk
- Sheep milk
- Buffalo milk
- Reindeer milk
- Jenny milk
- Dam milk

For example, buffalo milk is extensively used for the production of foods with notable historical traditions: the famous buffalo *mozzarella* cheese is the most known product for this category, despite the competition of another *mozzarella* cheese using cow milk curd [2]. On the other side, Italian *pecorino* cheeses are particularly appreciated because of the technology of production, while goat milk is well known and recommended for other reasons [3].

This chapter is explicitly dedicated to a little part of cow milk-derived products. In fact, cow milk is the most used ingredient for the production of cheeses in comparison with other milk [4].

Secondly, it should be noted that the different types of milk have strong influence on the technology and properties of final products, especially cheeses. Various factors have to be considered: initial chemical features, the typology of collection, the microbial ecology of the original milk. It is known [1] that ruminant mammals produce generally milk with notable amounts of proteins, including albumins, compared with other animals. This difference is important: in fact, the production of cheeses implies good textural properties for the final product, but this feature is strongly dependent on the quality and quantity of proteins. In other words, the higher the quantity and the molecular weight of proteins, caseins above all (these molecules are associations of different proteins), the higher the yield and textural properties of final cheeses. As a result, caseins appear the most important component in the production of cheeses.

With relation to cheeses, many important differences may be highlighted: the perspective of these milk-derived products may be very variegated [5].

From a general viewpoint, the whole group of cow milk-derived cheeses may be subdivided in the following way [1]:

(a) Fresh cheeses
(b) Soft cheeses
(c) Pressed cheeses
(d) *'Pasta filata'* cheeses
(e) Cheeses without coagulant agents (animal rennet, microbial enzymes, etc.)
(f) Cheeses from skimmed milk.

This classification corresponds to the viewpoint of the International Dairy Federation (IDF). The IDF has discriminated cheeses on the basis of a few known features [6]. However, other classifications may be proposed: the 'Codex General Standard for Cheese' is a useful example [7].

Anyway, all proposed classifications tend to be approximately similar by the chemical viewpoint: in fact, basic variables for chemical classification appear always the amount of moisture (and the consequent quantity of dry matter), the content of fat matter on the dry content, the 'moisture on free fat basis' (MFFB) index, the amount of salt (sodium chloride) on the dry content and pH values. The microbial ecology of cheeses and the technological process of production can be useful. For example, the following classifications appear mainly correlated to the technology of cheeses [8, 9]:

1. With reference to coagulation,

• Acid-coagulated cheeses
• Cheeses obtained by heat and acid at the same time
• Rennet-coagulated cheeses

2. With reference to texture,

- Extra-hard products
- Hard products
- Semi-hard products
- Soft cheeses

3. With relation to geographical origin,

- Dutch-type cheeses
- Swiss-type cheeses

4. With concern to the technology of ripening,

- Cheeses ripened 'in brine' [10]
- Unripened *pasta filata* products
- Mould-ripened cheeses
- Blue cheeses
- Other ripened cheeses like *Tilsit* [11]

5. With relation to industrial processes,

- Dried, processed products and analogue cheeses.

The last point is interesting because of the numerical growth of different varieties with the declared or undeclared intention of imitating other cheeses. For example, 'analogue' or 'analog' cheeses are processed preparations obtained from the mixing and melting of different ingredients: rennet casein, butter, vegetable oils, water, melting agents, colourants, etc. Most known products of this category seem to be [12]:

(a) Low-moisture *mozzarella* cheeses
(b) Normal and pasteurised processed cheddar
(c) Monterey jack.

Generally, processing techniques are similar to the usual method for obtaining pasteurised processed cheeses [13], except for the composition: processed products contain essentially cheeses with a small percentage of optional components and the exclusion of vegetable oils. These melted foods can represent a convenient option for cheesemakers: notable amounts of declassed cheese may be used and re-introduced in the so-called 'market flow', on condition that the food safety remains guaranteed with relation to final foods [14]. In addition, the re-use of declassed cheese has to be considered with the viewpoint of ISO 9001:2008-based quality systems. With reference to the food sector, two useful examples are the ISO 22000:2005 norm, the Global Standard for Food Safety (GSFS) and the International Featured Standards (IFS) Food. The quality of services and products, including 'ameliorated' versions, has to be adequately explained to the customer.

On the other side, there are different types of processed cheeses: one of these products, the 'dried' or 'powdered' cheese, is a fine-grained melted food with minimum moisture and good 'fat matter on dry content' values. Once more, many types of 'old' cheese or declassed products can be 'recycled' [14] with acceptable results from the chemical and microbiological viewpoint.

The aim of this chapter is the possibility of marking some 'analytical' line of discrimination between historical products and the heterogeneous group of modern industrial cheese, including 'cheese-like' products [12]. This study is important because of the economic implications (reduction of exercise expenses, increase of gross profits, etc.). On the other side, the production of 'ameliorated' versions of normal cheese should be considered based on the analytical viewpoint. Several hygienists could suppose these products correspond to the 'worsened' alternative of cheese: one of the possible objections could be the use of polyphosphates, according to Alais [1].

1.2 Ameliorated Versions of Artisanal Cheese: Economic Reasons and Other Advantages

The first reason for the increasing and diffused availability of cheese-like products appears related to the notable deficiency of raw materials in determined geographical areas. Moreover, the necessity of lowering exercise costs for the production of food preparations should be remembered. However, this approach may seem too simplified.

Many years ago, the exiguity or the complete lack of milk seemed to explain the strategy of cheesemakers: the use of imported raw materials for the production of cheese-like products. Moreover, the possible 'recycle' of hard cheese (swiss-type products, cheddar) as raw materials for the production of imitation cheeses seemed particularly interesting [1]. The chemical and technological explanation of these choices are simple enough: the melting procedure cannot give excellent results with high-moisture cheeses. In these products, casein molecules are generally similar to protein chains in the original milk: in other words, the hydrolytic breakdown of caseins into simpler and soluble fragments, proteose-peptones and amino acids is limited. As a result, mineral contents of caseins (calcium ions above all) remain high. On the one side, the abundance of calcium ions is absolutely needed in modern melting technologies if the aim is the increase of production yields [15, 16]. On the other side, calcium (Ca^{2+}) can act as chelating agent between different casein chains [17]: consequently, high Ca^{2+} contents may retard or make difficult the mixing of different cheeses with dissimilar proteolysis degrees. The presence of rennet casein [1, 15] in most formulations does not improve the situation because of the highest molecular weight (MW). Rennet casein can be intended as a mixture of different casein chains without a small polypeptide fraction [16–18].

As a result, the production of good or excellent processed cheeses would require the use of raw materials with several months of shelf life; seasoned cheeses (example: hard products) can be good ingredients. In seasoned products, casein chains should be short enough (low and very low MW) and the presence of Ca^{2+} ions should be numerically reduced because of the advanced proteolysis. The fusion at 100 °C or slightly lower temperatures [13] of similar cheeses with the addition of the right quantity of melting agents (polyphosphates, citrates) can be easily carried out. In fact, should Ca^{2+} ions be in excess, melting agents would replace this metal with sodium and the chelating effect of Ca^{2+} would disappear.

On the other hand, hard cheeses are not able to absorb water molecules like other products [19]. In fact, this property appears typical for high MW-casein chains with limited or absent proteolysis (examples: cow milk curds, *pasta filata* cheeses). For these reasons, processed cheeses with high shelf-life values should be produced with a good percentage of these 'soft' products.

Moreover, low or medium moisture cheeses have a common feature: the percentage of fat matter on the dry content can often reach 50 % and higher values [20, 21]. For this reason, cheese-like products have been progressively used for catering uses because of the predominant preference for soft and spicy tasted foods [15, 22]. With exclusive concern to sensorial features, the increase in the fat content determines the concomitant augment of the spicy or soft taste in cheeses with or without advanced fat fermentation by microbial lipases. A peculiar subcategory of cheese-like products comprehend analogue cheeses: the related formulation (water, seasoned and soft cheeses, vegetable oils, caseins, starches, colourants, hydrocolloids, preservatives, etc.) implies the same processing technique as melted cheeses [12], but final products may be realised with notable moisture contents (45–55 %).

The problem of moisture is directly correlated to the yield. In effect, the final amount of x Kg of cheese or cheese-like product may be different from the original sum of y Kg of used raw materials, including water. The quantity of absorbed water by rennet caseins and degraded cheeses (raw materials) depends on the average degree of proteolysis [16, 19]. Naturally, the addition of non-proteolysed rennet caseins is helpful because of their high absorption [15]. As a result, the higher the amount of non-proteolysed caseins, the higher the quantity of absorbed water in the melting process. Many components may have a role with reference to obtainable yields; several predictive equations might be useful for cheesemakers when speaking of normal cheeses and melted products.

Before continuing, it should be remembered that the economic convenience of cheese-like products has to be intended in terms of;

- Use of declassed cheeses or products with low economic value.
- Use of by-products of the milk and dairy industry.
- Possible addition of vegetable oils (related prices are normally lower if compared with animal butters).
- Possible management of aqueous absorption with consequent increase in yields.

1.3 The Theoretical Yield for Cheesemakers: The Fundamental Role of Rennet Caseins and Calcium Chloride

The yield depends on various factors: two of these variables are surely the quantity and the chemical composition of milk caseins. Actually, this name implies the existence of at least four different protein chains [1, 23]; these molecules are approximately 80 % of the total amount of proteins in cow milk.

First of all, it can be affirmed that the word 'casein' concerns all phosphoryl-ated proteins with the peculiar property of forming gels when the original milk is acidified at pH 4.6 [1]. Casein molecules can be easily separated from remaining serum proteins (albumins, globulins). Serum proteins can precipitate only under heating with limited applications for cheeses.

With relation to the group of casein molecules, it has to be highlighted that the proportion between basic atoms (carbon, hydrogen, oxygen, nitrogen) appears extremely constant in all discovered types [1]. The current subdivision concerns [24]:

1. α-casein. This name represents two different α_{s1} and α_{s2} types
2. β-casein. This substance and α-casein correspond to 70 % of the total casein amount; both proteins are able to form insoluble agglomerations in presence of Ca^{2+} ions
3. γ-casein. Actually, this name concerns three different molecules. Probably, they are fragments of β-casein
4. κ-casein. This protein (13 % of the total amount of caseins) is soluble at all possible temperatures on condition that Ca^{2+} ions are present. This compound is also responsible for the creation and the stabilisation of micellar suspensions in the original milk [23].

The separation between different caseins is not simple; in addition, there are no practical interests at present with concern to the production of peculiar casein types. As a consequence, the name 'casein' is currently used instead of the more correct distinction between known nitrogen-based molecules: α, β, γ and κ. This choice can be questionable from the analytical viewpoint but it can be used in simulated studies.

Another important feature of caseins is the notable amount of phosphorylated groups: their presence is useful because of the above-mentioned chelation effect between different protein chains, with the necessary presence of Ca^{2+} ions. In other words, the final yield is strongly dependent on the first step of cheesemak-ing: the production of the initial curd from the original milk. Chemically, this process corresponds to the coagulation and the precipitation of a heterogeneous matter from the original milk [1]. The coagulated matter is constituted of:

- 'Casein' molecules. Actually, the correct name should be 'paracasein' or 'para-κ-casein' [15, 24]
- Lipids, triglycerides above all. These esters, derived from glycerol and three fatty acids, are easily trapped [25] into the caseous agglomeration (insoluble and gelificated paracaseins, proteose-peptones, amino acids, etc.)
- Mineral salts. The prevailing cation is Ca^{2+} while phosphate groups are the most important fraction of electronegative ions [26]
- Water
- Carbohydrates (traces).

The coagulation of caseous matters is a three-step process: casein molecules are considered able to create stable molecular aggregates of colloidal size, also named micellar suspensions, because of the stabilising action of κ-casein.

The first step is the attack of κ-casein by chymosin or other coagulating enzymes. Attacked κ-casein is hydrolised with the detachment of a glycomacropeptide fraction

[4, 27, 28]. This simple reaction determines the collapse of existing micelles in the original milk and other casein types become free from chemical bonds and attractions. Should the presence of Ca^{2+} ions be abundant, a sort of chaotic agglomeration of different caseins would occur.

In detail, different protein chains tend to form a casein agglomeration or matrix around a hypothetical centre [29, 30]. The resulting gel network can easily avoid the migration of incorporated non-protein molecules: lipids, carbohydrates, etc. [26, 31]. Secondly, casein chains are composed of different peptide groups with the possibility of attracting water molecules by means of hydrogen bonds. Actually, the absorption can be limited [19] depending on the amount and disposition of triglycerides and partially demolished fat chains into the forming curd [25]. Moreover, another important factor has to be discussed.

The problem of the aqueous absorption is the main factor affecting cheesemaking yields [4, 16, 32]. In fact, the initial quantity of water molecules into the casein matrix depends on the degree of proteolysis: the higher the amount of fragmented casein chains, the lower the absorbed water despite peptide groups being free enough to move and search for thermodynamically favoured sterical dispositions [18, 19]. In a second step, the absorbed water is partially expelled from the gel network (syneresis): the paracasein network rearranges and contracts itself with the consequent expulsion of water in excess, serum proteins, nitrogen-based fractions and other little compounds [33, 34].

Finally, the remaining amount of absorbed water may be expelled in the final ripening step (actually, several cheeses do not need to be ripened). Moreover, an additional quantity of water is continually generated by hydrolysis because of the constant microbiological activity and other chemical reactions on proteins, lipids and remaining carbohydrates. On the other hand, unripened cheeses and packaged products without possibility of aqueous expulsion tend to show the apparent increase of the aqueous amount [18, 20]. Actually, the analytical increase is referred to moisture: this parameter is not coincident with the aqueous content. In addition, pH values and redox potentials tend to increase at the same time. Once more, main reasons are the constant microbiological activity and other chemical reactions on proteins, lipids and remaining carbohydrates.

With reference to cheesemaking yields, the result is influenced by the content and the chemical composition (MW, length of chains, number of peptide groups) of caseins. Moreover, the addition of calcium chloride ($CaCl_2$) in the process is important because of the increase in the coagulation speed until a certain level $CaCl_2$ is normally added with coagulating enzymes and its role can be explained in the following way [1, 34]:

(a) pH values are normally lowered in cow milk if amino acids and phosphate groups into caseins lose progressively their protons with the subsequent substitution by Ca^{2+} ions. As a result, measurable reductions in rennet gelation times (RGT) have been observed with the concomitant increase of curd firming rate and firmness. However, RGT seem to decrease if the addition of $CaCl_2$ remains between 2 and 9 mMol because Ca^{2+} in excess tend to react with negatively charged carboxyl groups on caseins

(b) The average dimension of micellar suspensions appears to increase with the
    addition of $CaCl_2$, while caseins seems to prefer the micellar disposition
    instead of the soluble form.

As a consequence, added $CaCl_2$ may increase cheesemaking yields: in fact, different para-κ-casein chains tend to form stable ionic bonds by means of the presence
of Ca^{2+} ions between peptide groups in the enolic disposition [1]. For this reason,
analytical reports for different cheeses may show higher Ca^{2+} values compared
with the scientific literature [15, 35]. On the other hand, $CaCl_2$ is widely used for
the production of various dairy products: for example, rennet caseins for food
grade applications can be cited.

   However, the natural detection of Ca^{2+} in normal milks may give a peculiar difficulty with concern to the production of cheese-like products: the necessary reduction of this element in excess with sequestrating agents (polyphosphates, citrates
and other additives). The result should be the substitution of Ca^{2+} with sodium and
the consequent reduction of calcium phosphate crosslinks between para-κ-casein
molecules [13]; in addition, the aqueous absorption should be easier.

   Substantially, the addition of $CaCl_2$ is important because of the increase in the
amount of coagulated caseins and lipids (these chains are entrapped into the gel
network). However, the aqueous absorption is not directly influenced by the presence of Ca^{2+} ions. In effect, the cheesemaking yield can be intended in two different ways:

1. The production of a specified amount of curd from the original milk.
2. The production of cheeses and cheese-like products by complex formulations;
   for example, 'low moisture' *mozzarella* cheeses [36].

With reference to the normal concept of cheesemaking yield, this quantity can be
defined as the amount of produced cheese in kg from 100 kg of milk [36]. Other
authors prefer to describe yields as the number of kilograms of produced cheese
from 100 l of milk [16]. It has to be noted that other formulations can be proposed:
the 'moisture-adjusted cheese' yield or the percentage of fat recovered in cheese
[31]. The real hope of cheesemakers is the possibility of predicting one of these
yields on the basis of a few parameters, in spite of the variability of original milks
[16]. Normally, most known and used predictive equations consider the influence
of fat and casein amounts of the original milk [4]. The general equation is:

$$CY = aF + bC + e \qquad (1.1)$$

where a and b are dependent on the influence of fat and casein contents on the
cheesemaking yield (CY). In addition, e is a constant, dependent on the loss of
casein and the amount of non-fat and non-casein solid matters in the final cheese.
Actually, e may be 0 [4].

   Van Slyke's equation and related modifications for cheddar cheeses can also be
mentioned: the interested reader is invited to read other literature works. However,
obtainable results should be validated for every cheese type and production [4].

   Another recent study has been published [16, 22, 37] with reference to the cal-
culation of cheesemaking yields. This approach—the 'Cheesemaking Yield and

Proteins Estimation according to Parisi:2006' (CYPEP:2006) indirect method—can be used for the determination of yields and the most reliable amount of proteins in cheeses. Two similar free software, the Compact Cheese Spreadsheets (CCS), versions 1.0 and 1.1 [37] and the SynCheese Suite 2009 [38], have been realised on the basis of CYPEP:2006.

The CYPEP:2006 approach can be helpful for the determination of different cheesemaking yields from the original milk, but other applications may be interesting with reference to cheese-like products. Section 1.4 shows several of these applications.

1.4 A Predictive Equation for the Calculation of the Theoretical Yield: Analogue Cheeses

Generally, cheesemaking yields can be predicted on the basis of main chemical data of the original milk [1]. This approach is justified when speaking of 'pure' cheeses from milk, salt and rennet only, but modern cheesemakers would need to obtain reliable data and predictions for the production of industrial imitation cheeses. This necessity is particularly important if the final production of processed cheeses is very far from the geographical location of the milk collection and the intermediate storage [21].

In addition, the yield of normal cheeses from 'ready-to-use' curds should be predicted depending on features of the designed product. In other words, the use of ready curds from different locations can give several problems because this type of raw material may be unable to absorb more water in subsequent steps. As a consequence, reliable cheesemaking yields could be better calculated when following cheese parameters are known before the production:

- Moisture content (MC) or dry matter (DM), and
- Fat content on dry matter (FDM).

These data are well known in the cheesemaking industry and easily calculable.

The above-mentioned CYPEP:2006 method is based on these two data [16]. It has to be noted this procedure is available in two different versions: in fact, the 'rigorous and corrected' (R&C) method may sometimes give incorrect or incompatible results because of peculiar preconditions [37]. For this reason, a second and 'rapid' approach is available: this version can furnish slightly different results if compared with the R&C approach, but related differences are acceptable. In addition, the rapid approach can also be used for calculating related errors.

The basic aim of the CYPEP:2006 method is the reliable prediction of the theoretical CY (Kg/10 l of milk). At the same time, the most probable amount of proteins in the final cheese may be calculated: however, this content is the quantity of nitrogen in grams multiplied 6.38 (milk and milk-based products) instead of the currently accepted conversion factor for proteins in foods (6.25). The basic equation (R&C approach) is [16, 18]:

$$CY = \frac{MC}{MFFB} \times 2.47 + 6.98 \qquad (1.2)$$

This equation is mainly based on the quantity 'MC/MFFB': the minimum CY should be 6.98 kg/100 l of milk if MC (and the resulting MC/MFFB ratio) = 0. On the basis of the prediction of CY, other data can be obtained by means of CYPEP:2006 in both rigorous and rapid procedures [16]:

• Presumptive 'high-adsorption' casein (CAS_{HA}). This quantity corresponds to the undemolished 'casein' with high water absorption (estimated MW: 22,296 Da). CAS_{HA} is a simulated casein molecule with an average MW between different casein types. It can be obtained by means of the following equation:

•

$$CAS_{HA} = CY \times \frac{21.6}{12.5} \qquad (1.3)$$

• Presumptive 'high-absorption' pre-casein (p-CAS_{HA}). This quantity is the undemolished 'casein' with low water absorption (estimated MW > 22,296 Da). It can be found in curds with limited protein degradation and highest Ca^{2+} content. p-CAS_{HA} corresponds to a simulated casein molecule with low hydric absorption compared with CAS_{HA}. Chemically, p-CAS_{HA} is different from CAS_{HA} for the presence of the original glycomacropeptide. This fraction is removed after the primary hydrolytic reaction by means of the chymosin action
• The 'most reliable amount' (MRA) of proteins in cheeses (TP_{MRA}). According to the rapid version of CYPEP:2006, $TP_{MRA} = MFFB \times 0.84$
• Apparent hydric absorption (A%). By the mathematical viewpoint, A% is equal to (CAS_{HA}/TP_{MRA}) × 100. Two different situations can occur:

  – A% represents the hydric adsorption of caseins when the cheese structure corresponds to one solid and diphasic system: 'water, caseins and other dissolved substances' (aqueous phase) and 'fat matter' (organic phase). In this situation, A% may reach 100 %
  – A% may also mean the hydric adsorption of caseins when the cheese structure is done by the coexistence of:

    1. One solid and diphasic system: 'water, caseins and other dissolved substances' (aqueous phase) and 'fat matter' (organic phase), and
    2. A second liquid phase (water) that can be considered 'totally free' and continually relocated inside the solid diphasic matrix. In this situation, A% exceeds 100 %

All above-mentioned definitions may be helpful with relation to the chemistry and technology of cheeses [25]: the nature of analogue cheeses may be studied with this simulative approach.

1.5 Peculiar Properties of Analogue Cheeses and Related Explanation by Means of the CYPEP:2006 Method

A simulative study of the composition and properties of analogue cheeses is shown here. In detail, this example concerns the composition of a peculiar product obtained with the following list of ingredients: water, rennet casein, vegetable oils, butter, cheeses, citric acid (acidity corrector) and sodium citrate (melting agent). Similar processed foods have been studied in recent years [15, 20, 21].

The following data are known for the above-mentioned analogue cheese, version 1:

- MC = 52.2 %
- FC = 20.5 %.

On these bases, other data can be calculated by means of CYPEP:2006 or the CCS:

- The MFFB index. This number (65.7 %) can be correlated to firmness and ripening features of cheeses [3]
- The theoretical yield (naturally, this number is without real meaning here because processed cheeses are not directly obtained from milk). With reference to our situation, CY = 11.7 kg per 100 l
- The apparent hydric absorption (A%). For this cheese, A% = 88.2 %.

On the basis of these results, it can be inferred that:

1. The designed product should be soft enough: MFFB value for soft cheeses is normally higher than 67 % according to the CODEX STAN 283-1978 document [7]
2. CY may be useful to our situation in spite of the nature of analogue cheeses. Should the above calculated data be referred to a 'true' cheese (obtained by milk, salt and rennet only), it would be affirmed that the related cheesemaking yield has been 'high' [1]. In other words, obtained cheeses should give good prices from the economic viewpoint. On the other hand, it could be affirmed that the analogue cheese-like product is economically interesting in comparison to other similar processed products because of high CY values.

Finally, A% = 88.2 % means that 88.2 % of the MRA quantity of proteins can absorb the maximum water content because of the status of non-proteolysed caseins. In other words, the molecular profile of these proteins should show a peculiar abundance of high-MW-casein chains. This molecular profile can be shown by means of CCS: this free software can display a diagram of different MW (Fig. 1.1) and the non-proteolysed fraction is on the right of the diagram.

In contrast, most proteolysed caseins, proteose-peptones, other protein traces and simple amino acids (low MW) are progressively displayed from the left to the centre (MW = 11,148 Da) of the diagram. These molecules remain constantly under A% = 5 %, while a notable fraction between the centre and the right of the diagram shows A% ≥ 5 %.

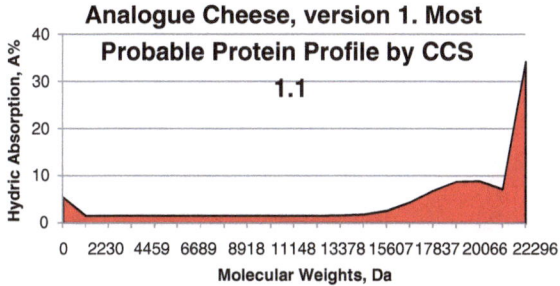

Fig. 1.1 The most probable profile of proteins for the first version of an analogue cheese according to CCS, version 1.1. This diagram shows the non-proteolysed fraction of caseins on the *right* (high MW) with the highest value of A%, and another area with low A% between MW = 18,952 and 20,066 Da. Degraded casein chains (proteolysed caseins, protease-peptones, other protein traces and simple amino acids) are progressively displayed from the *left* of the diagram (low MW, low A%) to the centre (MW = 11,148 Da; A% < 5 %)

This simulation may help cheese technologists with possible amelioration of the product in the design step. For example, the analogue cheese may be realised with more firmness: mathematically, this would mean that MFFB has to be lowered. As a consequence, the resulting product should give lower prices compared with the first version because of CY and A% values. A possible solution may be the design of another 'version 2' with the same MC content and FC = 15.0 %.

Consequently, CYPEP:2006 and CCS would calculate the following new values:

- MFFB = 61.4 % (it was 65.7 % for version 1)
- CY = 10.9 kg per 100 l (it was 11.7 for version 1)
- A% = 68.4 % (it was 88.2 % for version 1).

Yield values for versions 1 and 2 are similar, but the difference between A% numbers is notable (19.8 %). In addition, the diagram of the most probable protein profile can be shown for the second version (Fig. 1.2).

Figure 1.2 shows that the highest peak on the right side- CAS_{HA}—does not reach 25 % (it was 35 % in Fig. 1.1), while the extreme left peak is notably increased. From the chemical viewpoint, the following interpretation can be expressed: version 2 contains more proteolysed proteins from 'old' cheeses (raw materials) compared with the amount of added rennet caseins, and A% has been naturally lowered. At the same time, the final product can be firmer than the initial version; this implies also the augment of chewiness. On the other side, the increase in CY is moderate (+6.8 % in comparison with the original value).

Finally, cheese technologists could desire to create softer products than the original version 1. Should this be the main goal, the FC value would necessarily be increased. For example, the new analogue cheese (version 3) may be realised with the same MC content and FC = 26.0 %. Consequently, CYPEP:2006 and CCS would calculate the following values:

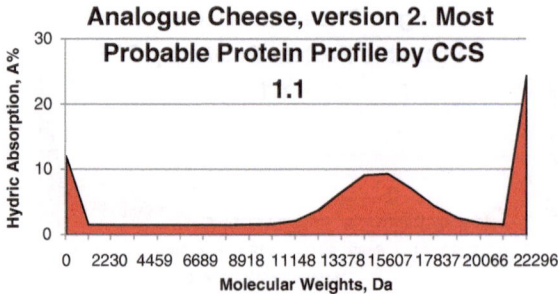

Fig. 1.2 The most probable profile of proteins for the second version of an analogue cheese according to CCS, version 1.1. This diagram shows the non-proteolysed fraction of caseins on the *right* (high MW) with the highest value of A%, and another important area with low A% between MW = 14,492 and 15,607 Da. Degraded casein chains (proteolysed caseins, proteose-peptones, other protein traces and simple amino acids) are progressively displayed from the *left* of the diagram (low MW, A% > 10 %) to the centre (MW = 11,148 Da; A% < 5 %)

- MFFB = 70.5 % (it was 65.7 % for version 1)
- CY = 12.9 kg per 100 l (it was 11.7 for version 1)
- A% = 121.7 % (it was 88.2 % for version 1).

The new analogue cheese is certainly softer than the original product; in addition, yields and the capability of absorbing water by caseins seem to be enhanced. On the other hand, the economic value of these products may be low. This commercial and technological concept seems in contrast with the above shown conclusions.

In effect, the opinion of technologist is referred to (a) the mathematical result of cheese processing and (b) the production of good products with relation to the acceptability of shelf life and technological properties (chewiness, firmness, melting,…), including quality parameters.

According to CYPEP:2006, CY and A% increased values demonstrate that the original version may be modified with the desired augment of the final quantity of cheese. This approach also means that the final cheese-like product contains too much water with reference to the amount of high-absorption caseins: A% > 100 %.

From the chemical viewpoint, the exceeding water can be imagined as a liquid-like fraction in contact with the solid and diphasic cheese [19]: water molecules are weakly linked with casein peptide groups by means of hydrogen bonds, but there are two additional aqueous layers between proteins and the liquid-like phase. In other words, every peptide group can establish up to four different hydrogen bonds with water, but the upper aqueous layer can create hydrogen bonds with other molecules. This structure corresponds to a double-layered network of water around proteins: the first layer, strongly connected to caseins, might be roughly identified with the 'linked water', while the second layer is a notable part or the totality of 'free water'. Finally, there is the possibility of connecting the second aqueous layer with other water, if available: the resulting third layer is continually connected and relocated on the surface of the second layer because of the intrinsic

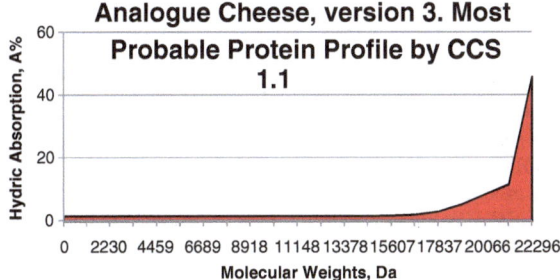

Fig. 1.3 The most probable profile of proteins for the third version of an analogue cheese according to CCS, version 1.1. This diagram shows the non-proteolysed fraction of caseins on the *right* (high MW) with A% > 45 %. This time, the most part of caseins appears substantially circumscribed between MW = 18,952 and 22,296 Da; A% is ≥5 %. On the other side, most degraded casein chains (MW ≤ 11,148 Da) are not abundant. This fraction remains constantly under A% < 5 %

weakness of hydrogen bonds between water molecules. The exceeding water can also temporarily enter the casein network.

As a result, the designed cheese would show peculiar features: '*mozzarella* cheese in water' is surely one of cheeses with this behaviour. This product is well known for the property of releasing drops of absorbed water: this water corresponds to the above-mentioned third layer. From the mathematical viewpoint, the apparent hydric absorption is higher than 100.

Figure 1.3 shows the most probable protein profile for version 3: the extreme right peak- CAS_{HA}—has increased the related abundance, while the extreme left peak does not reach A% = 5 %. In other words, most part of the proteins (18.3 %, according to CYPEP:2006) correspond to CAS_{HA} (more rennet caseins, reduced quantity of 'old' cheeses in the formula) and the related absorption is really enhanced.

At the same time, the final product is surely softer than version 1 and there is the possibility of seeing aqueous drops emerging from the cheese surface at room temperature. This expulsive phenomenon is caused by the temporary absorption of water in excess. These molecules are not directly linked to proteins because of their localisation in the third layer; their distance from peptide groups is notable [19].

Consequently, cheese technologists have to make their choice: on the one side, the increase in CY and the concomitant reduction of costs; on the other hand, the production of long shelf-life products with reduced moisture, enhanced firmness and ameliorated technological features (chewiness, slicing, etc.).

Similar examples may help readers to learn several aspects of the production and correlated strategies in the market of analogue cheeses and cheese-like products.

References

1. Alais C (1984) Science du lait. Principles des techniques laitières, 4th edn. S.E.P.A.I.C., Paris
2. Gobbetti M (2007) What is a controlled designation of origin? In: McSweeney PLH (ed) Cheese problems solved. Woodhead Publishing Limited, Cambridge, pp. 178–180
3. Park YW (2009) Bioactive components in goat milk. In: Park YW (ed) Bioactive components in milk and dairy products. John Wiley & Sons Inc., New York, pp 43–81
4. Banks JM (2007) Why is ultrafiltration used for cheesemaking and how is it applied? In: McSweeney PLH (ed) Cheese problems solved. Woodhead Publishing Limited, Cambridge, pp 30–33
5. Ottogalli G (2001) Atlante dei formaggi. Ulrico Hoepli Editore, Milan
6. Burkhalter G (1981) Catalogue of Cheeses. International Dairy Federation, Brussels
7. Codex Alimentarius Commission (1978) Codex Stan 283-1978: general standard for cheese, rev.1-1999, amd.3-2008. Codex Alimentarius—International Food Standards, Rome
8. McSweeney PLH (2007) Principal families of cheese. In: McSweeney PLH (ed) Cheese problems solved. Woodhead Publishing Limited, Cambridge, pp 176–177
9. McSweeney PLH, Ottogalli G, Fox PF (2004) Diversity of cheese varieties: an overview. In: Fox PF, McSweeney PLH, Cogan TM, Guinee TP (eds) Cheese: chemistry, physics and microbiology, vol 2, 3rd edn. Elsevier Academic Press, Amsterdam, pp 1–22
10. Codex Alimentarius Commission (1999) Codex Stan 208-1999: Codex Group Standard for Cheeses in Brine, amd. 2010. Codex Alimentarius—International Food Standards, Rome
11. McSweeney PLH (2007) Introduction: what are bacterial surface-ripened (smear) cheeses? In: McSweeney PLH (ed) Cheese problems solved. Woodhead Publishing Limited, Cambridge, pp 289–290
12. Guinee TP (2007) Introduction: what are analogue cheeses? In: McSweeney PLH (ed) Cheese problems solved. Woodhead Publishing Limited, Cambridge, pp 384–386
13. Guinee TP (2007) Introduction: what is processed cheese? In: McSweeney PLH (ed) Cheese problems solved. Woodhead Publishing Limited, Cambridge, pp 365–367
14. Food Standards Agency (2007) Cheese recovery guidance. Food Standards Agency, London
15. Parisi S (2006) Profili chimici delle caseine presamiche alimentari. IndAliment 457:377–383
16. Parisi S, Laganà P, Delia AS (2006) Il calcolo indiretto del tenore proteico nei formaggi: il metodo CYPEP. IndAliment 462:997–1010
17. Udabage P, McKinnon IR, Augustin MA (2000) Mineral and casein equilibria in milk: effects of added salts and calcium-chelating agents. J Dairy Res 67:361–370
18. Parisi S, Laganà P, Delia AS (2007) Lo studio dei profili proteici durante la maturazione dei formaggi tramite il metodo CYPEP. IndAliment 468:404–417
19. Parisi S, Laganà P, Stilo A, Micali M, Piccione D, Delia S (2009) Il massimo assorbimento idrico nei formaggi. Tripartizione del contenuto acquoso per mole d'azoto. IndAliment 491:31–41
20. Parisi S (2002) Profili evolutivi dei contenuti batterici e chimico-fisici in prodotti lattiero-caseari. IndAliment 412:295–306
21. Parisi S (2003) Evoluzione chimico-fisica e microbiologica nella conservazione di prodotti lattiero-caseari. IndAliment 423:249–259
22. Parisi S (2012) Food packaging and food alterations: the user-oriented approach. SmithersRapra Technology, Shawbury
23. Kelly AL (2007) Milk. What is the typical composition of cow's milk and what milk constituents favour cheesemaking? In: McSweeney PLH (ed) Cheese problems solved. Woodhead Publishing Limited, Cambridge, pp 3–4
24. McSweeney PLH (2007) Introduction: how does rennet coagulate milk? In: McSweeney PLH (ed) Cheese problems solved. Woodhead Publishing Limited, Cambridge, pp 50–51
25. Parisi S, Caruso G (2013) Il regolamento CE 2073/2005 e successivi aggiornamenti. Studio di piani di campionamento ridotti per formaggi molli altamente deperibili. Ind Aliment (in press)

26. McSweeney PLH (2007) Milk. Introduction. In: McSweeney PLH (ed) Cheese problems solved. Woodhead Publishing Limited, Cambridge, pp 1–2

27. Kelly AL (2007) What are milk salts and how do they affect the properties of cheese? In: McSweeney PLH (ed) Cheese problems solved. Woodhead Publishing Limited, Cambridge, pp 7–8

28. O'Mahony JA, Lucey JA, McSweeney PLH (2005) Chymosin-mediated proteolysis, calcium solubilisation and texture development during the ripening of Cheddarcheese. J Dairy Sci 88:3101–3114. doi:10.3168/jds.S0022-0302(05)72992-1

29. Guinee TP (2007) What effects does cold storage have on the properties of milk? In: McSweeney PLH (ed) Cheese problems solved. Woodhead Publishing Limited, Cambridge, pp 28–29

30. Fox PF, McSweeney PLH (1998) Dairy chemistry and biochemistry. Blackie Academic and Professional, London

31. Banks JM (2007) How can cheese yield be predicted? In: McSweeney PLH (ed) Cheese problems solved. Woodhead Publishing Limited, Cambridge, pp 105–106

32. McSweeney PLH (2007) Introduction: what is syneresis? In: McSweeney PLH (ed) Cheese problems solved. Woodhead Publishing Limited, Cambridge, pp 72–73

33. Dejmek P, Walstra P (2004) The syneresis of rennet-coagulated curd. In: Fox PF, McSweeney PLH, Cogan TM, Guinee TP (eds) Cheese: chemistry, physics and microbiology, vol 1, 3rd edn. Elsevier Academic Press, Amsterdam, pp 71–103

34. Fox PF, Guinee TP, McSweeney PLH, Cogan TM (eds) (2000) Fundamentals of cheese science. Aspen, Gaithersburg

35. O'Brien NM, O'Connor TP (2004) Nutritional aspects of cheese. In: Fox PF, McSweeney PLH, Cogan TM, Guinee TP (eds) Cheese: chemistry, physics and microbiology vol 1, 3rd edn. Elsevier Academic Press, Amsterdam, pp 573–581

36. Banks JM (2007) How is cheese yield defined? In: McSweeney PLH (ed) Cheese problems solved. Woodhead Publishing Limited, Cambridge, pp 102–104

37. Parisi S (2010) Compact CheeseSpreadsheets: software per l'analisi delle proteine nei formaggi. IndAliment 498:50–51

38. Parisi S, Delia S, Cannavò G, Pino R, Mauro A, Laganà P (2009) Validazione della raccolta software SynCheese Suite 2009, versione 1.0, per il calcolo di vari parametri analitici dei formaggi. Relazioni tra assorbimento idrico e alterazione microbiologica dei formaggi confezionati. Ig Sanità Pubbl 5/2009, supplement, p 394

39. Kindstedt PS (2007) What are pasta-filata cheeses and what physicochemical changes occur during cooking/stretching? In: McSweeney PLH (ed) Cheese problems solved. Woodhead Publishing Limited, Cambridge, pp 300–301

40. Parisi S (2013) Food industry and packaging materials—performance-oriented guidelines for users. SmithersRapra Technology, Shawbury

Chapter 2
The Prediction of Shelf Life Values in Function of the Chemical Composition in Soft Cheeses

Abstract The determination of shelf life of food products is one of the most important problems in the modern industry. With reference to this argument, the list of scientific papers is long enough. It should be considered that the food production is subdivided into a number of different fields and subsectors, depending on the typology of raw materials, intermediates, finished products and by-products. In addition, every class of food product can be easily expanded in comparison with the classification of the Codex Alimentarius Commission due to the presence of industrial imitations. Several of these industrial products may be perceived as 'ameliorated' versions of the original prototype. The prediction of food durability is certainly influenced by several parameters: the typology of process, the packaging system, the choice of the correct storage condition and other factors. Moreover, the function of food additives should be discussed. The food producer is always responsible for the correctness of nutritional data and other information related to the food product, including the durability. The aim of this paper is to review previous theories and related calculations for the preventive determination of shelf life values in cheeses, especially soft products. These calculations are based on the approximate chemical formulation of the final product. Authors have also discussed the possible modification of predictive equations for a peculiar *pasta filata* product, the so-called '*mozzarella* cheese in water'.

Keywords Casein · Hydrolysis · Moisture · *Mozzarella* cheese · Shelf life · Yeasts and moulds

2.1 The Food Durability: An Overview

The determination of shelf life (SL) of food products is one of the most important problems in the modern industry. With reference to this argument, the list of scientific papers is long enough [1, 2].

It should be considered that the food production is subdivided in a number of different fields and subsectors, depending on the typology of raw materials,

G. Barbieri et al., *The Influence of Chemistry on New Foods and Traditional Products*, Chemistry of Foods, DOI 10.1007/978-3-319-11358-6_2

intermediates, finished products and by-products. In addition, every class of food product can be easily expanded in comparison with the classification of the Codex Alimentarius Commission [3] because of the presence of industrial imitations. Moreover, several of these industrial products may be often perceived as 'ameliorated' versions of the original prototype by consumers [4–7].

The prediction of food durability is influenced by several parameters: the typology of process [8], the packaging material and related packing systems [9], the choice of the correct storage condition [8] and other factors. In addition, the function of food additives should be considered [10]. The food producer is always responsible for the correctness of nutritional data and other information related to the food product, including the durability.

The aim of this paper is to review several theories and related calculations for the preventive determination of SL values in cheeses, especially soft products. These calculations are based on the approximate chemical formulation of the final product. Moreover, the possible modification of predictive equations has been discussed for a peculiar type of *pasta filata* product, '*mozzarella* cheese in water'.

From a general viewpoint, it can be affirmed that the SL of foods and beverages is strictly related to the typology of food product; on these bases, food durability may be considered as a sort of 'fingerprint' for the peculiar food and might be used for identification and classification purposes. Two or more similar products may have the same SL; consequently, the concept of 'fingerprint' may be questionable [8]. On the other hand, the SL may be considered as a performance indicator for foods and beverages. In effect, the simple colorimetric modification of certain products may signal that the related food is or appears expired [9, 11]. As a result, the exact determination of the temporal period between the production of foods and the 'unacceptable' modification of sensorial features may be expressed as a simple number: in other words, every food may be classified by means of this 'performance value' [9, 12]. According to the 'principle of food degradation' [8], all edible products are exposed to the continuous and unstoppable transformation of chemical, physical, microbiological and technological features during time, in all possible storage conditions.

Moreover, the estimation of food durability values needs solid mathematical bases because the 'true' SL has to be centred into a numerical range with maximum and minimum limits [13]. However, this requirement—the existence of mathematical restrictions—might be the cause of problems when related equations have to be solved and obtained results have to be verified in the real world. One of the most interesting approaches may be the predictive estimation of a minimum SL with accessory 'positive' errors [1]. On these bases, the minimum SL would be always reliable while the mathematical error should influence only the maximum value.

The following list contains main factors affecting SL values:

(a) Food or beverage type (category). Examples: meat and meat-based products; fruits and vegetables; milk and milk products; seafood; industrial preparations
(b) Food or beverage sub-class. A useful reference is the 'Codex General Standard for Food Additives', Annex B, Parts I and II [3]

(c) Processing technology, from raw materials to finished products
(d) Packaging procedures, including the preliminary evaluation of packaging materials
(e) Storage conditions with peculiar reference to temperatures and logistics
(f) Every parameter (microbiological counts, chemical contents, etc.) with influence on sensory features of food products.

From a general viewpoint, the problem of the correct and reliable determination of SL values may be difficult and 'thorny'; related responsibilities are ascribed to the food producer [13].

In detail, the determination of food durability values can be complex because of a number of different factors; the subdivision of foods and beverages in peculiar categories is helpful. A typical example is related to the production of cheeses: with concern to these products, SL depends basically on the following points [14]:

- Cleaning methods and sanitisation procedures for pipelines and milk collection equipment.
- The chemical and microbiological condition of used raw milks.
- Storage conditions, with peculiar reference to thermal values.

The 'Hazard Analysis and Critical Control Points' (HACCP) approach implies that the production of hygienically sure and compliant foods cannot be demonstrated when the above-mentioned basic information and other data are not considered by cheesemakers [15].

Other important points are:

- The influence of food packaging materials (FPM) on the SL of the packaged cheese [16, 17]
- The use of food additives, antimicrobial agents and other chemicals for production of 'ameliorated' and 'imitation' cheeses. For example several additives—nisin, sodium propionate, potassium sorbate—may be used because of their notable action against moulds in analogue products [7].

However, the category of cheeses may appear extremely variegated and the determination of food durability values cannot be discussed from a general viewpoint. As a result, authors have decided to mention the peculiar class of 'pasta filata' products and the related sub-category of mozzarella cheeses (MZR) with the aim of giving useful demonstrations and examples. In addition, abundant scientific literature is available about mozzarella cheeses.

2.2 Cheeses and Food Durability

The category of pasta filata cheeses is included in the general macrogroup of rennet-coagulated cheeses [5]: this list concerns 10 different cheese subclasses at least. One of the main features of pasta filata cheeses is substantially related to the distribution of the amorphous 'paracasein': this name means a small group of milk proteins. Paracaseins are generally rearranged and aligned into roughly parallel fibres [18] by means of a peculiar technique of cheese production. In detail, the original raw milk (different types are used, but most known applications are related to cow's and buffalo's milks) is coagulated with the use of animal, vegetable or microbial enzymes to obtain the so-called 'curd'. This intermediate material is subsequently 'cooked and stretched' in hot water. The final result is a peculiar protein matrix containing also fat globules (variable dimensions). As a consequence, the heterogeneous quasi-laminar structure of caseins determines peculiar features of *pasta filata* cheeses. For example the exceptional stretchability is dependent on the behaviour of proteins. Caseins may be considered as organic textile fibres: consequently, should the curd be drawn in a single direction with the addition of hot water, these protein chains would easily dispose themselves in parallel and roughly ordered lines.

Naturally, good products need adequate raw materials and correct conditions: the right acidity of raw milks and the resulting curd, the correct quantity of calcium, the high water temperature and the speed of mixer screws [18].

The main and most known *pasta filata* product in the world is probably *mozzarella* cheese. A number of different versions and 'ameliorated' foods with this name are available at present. The low-moisture *mozzarella* cheese (LMMC) is a good example [18].

From the technical viewpoint, MZR are not ripened products [19]: these foods can be heated or used without other processes a few hours after the production. However, ripening modifications can occur in MZR during their SL period: in fact, it may be affirmed that *pasta filata* cheeses tend to change their original composition and the microbial population into the packaging container. This situation corresponds to a series of different reactions and microbial fermentations: normally, 'fresh' cheeses may show these anomalies when the related food durability exceeds 15 days.

For this and other reasons, microbiological limits for this type of cheese appear very rigorous: legally, the European Regulation (EC) No 2073/2005 and subsequent amendments has defined strict requirements. Another example can be shown: the french *Fédération des Entreprises du Commerce et de la Distribution* (FCD, French Retail and Wholesale Federation) has forced cheese producers to consider additional parameters with reference to unripened cheeses from pasteurised milk [20]. With reference to yeasts and moulds, the following rules are mandatory:

- 100 colony-forming units (CFU) per gram at the arrival near mass retailers.
- 100 CFU per gram at the end of SL periods (expiration or 'best before end' date).

These requirements, valuable for French mass retailers only, are not absolute: yeasts and moulds can reach 5,000 CFU/g at the reception near mass retailers for *mozzarella* and similar traditional cheeses, while 50,000 CFU/g can be tolerated at the end of SL [20].

This simple example shows how the management of *pasta filata* cheeses may be difficult from the microbiological viewpoint. Basically, the FCD recognises that the limit of yeasts and moulds may notably increase. As an implicit result, SL values can be dependent on the variable behaviour of these life forms into cheeses.

Moreover, the peculiar subclass of MZR is composed of various versions: there is no real possibility of defining one SL value only for all existing products with this name. For example, the same *mozzarella* cheese can be packed into plastic containers of different types with or without water: the first group concerns products with notable weights (400- 1,000–2,000 g, etc.), while the second category is normally produced as little spheres ('cherries') with reduced weight: 5, 6, 8, 10, 100 or 250 g. It has to be highlighted that these two classes of *mozzarella* cheese show dissimilar behaviours during their SL. Naturally, the microbial spreading should be easily predicted and notably accelerated when cheeses are immersed in water, and the possible modification of sensorial features is further increased because of the small dimension of products (lower weights = higher contact surface between cheeses and water). Additionally, yeasts and moulds are non-pathogenic agents but cheeses can be excellent 'culture media' for different degrading life forms [1]: this risk has to be carefully taken into account when speaking of cheeses in water.

2.3 Soft Cheeses and Cherries in Water: Predictable Differences

As above mentioned, the group of *pasta filata* cheeses comprehends different products: most known cheeses are *mozzarella*, *provolone*, *kashkaval* [4, 21] and *halloumi* [22]. MZR are particularly studied because of the absence of ripening periods. However, several modifications—hydrolysis, expulsion of proteolysed substances and fatty molecules dissolved in water, enhanced fermentation by *Lactobacillaceae* and *Streptococcae*, microbial spreading—may occur within 15 days after the initial production into the final packaging [23].

When MZR are packed without water, the sum of the above-mentioned transformations can be easily identified with a sort of undesired 'maturation' of the initial cheese into the container. The casein matrix tends to remove the exceeding water (the original aqueous content and the result of the additional hydrolysis) and different dissolved molecules: calcium and sodium salts, proteose-peptones, organic acids (by microbial fermentation), etc. It has to be noted that this exceeding water is not allowed to drain unless perforated packages are used. Consequently, packaged MZR are essentially metastable products because of the presence of contaminated and exceeding hydrolysis water at the food/packaging interface. Generally, MZR tend to show excessive softness [24] with reference to external layers of the product (surfaces are clearly the softest section). In addition, pH values tend to increase and oxidation-reduction (redox) potentials may turn to negative values [25]. The same phenomenon has been observed in different cheeses produced from sheep milk [26, 27].

As a consequence, the microbial spreading by yeasts and other degrading life forms can become important because of one or more of the following conditions:

• Negative values of redox potentials.
• Increase of water and degraded substances.

Should this situation be observed, the packaged *mozzarella* cheese would become superficially degraded and non-edible: in other words, an unpredictable reduction of the declared SL would be noted [1].

Apparently, the above described phenomenon might appear 'silent' when speaking of MZR in water. For example, *mozzarella* cherries in water show a peculiar behaviour. In detail, this product is initially able to absorb a certain amount of 'external' water into the packaging material [28] depending on:

• The degree of proteolysis of para-κ-caseins (Sect. 1.3), and
• The fat content on dry matter (FDM) amount [29].

As a clear and macroscopic consequence, MZR tends to increase their weight compared with the initial value. Modest dimensions of cheese spheres (cherries) are also a distinctive advantage: the higher the global surface (cheeses are subdivided in small pieces), the higher the observable absorption.

This important step should occur on the first day after the initial production. However, high FDM values or advanced proteolysis can diminish the predictable absorption of water. Subsequently, *mozzarella* cherries tend to release progressively water. As above mentioned, this water is composed of two fractions:

1. The initial absorbed water on the first day after the final packaging (variable amount) and the original aqueous amount of cheeses.
2. The total quantity of exceeding water (cause: partially degraded caseins become more and more unable to absorb water depending on the degree of proteolysis and the reduction of molecular weights).

Additionally, the microbial spreading is really enhanced in the external and constantly wetted layers of *mozzarella* cherries. The visual detection of spoiled MZR may be difficult because of non-transparent packages and the suspension in water. On the other hand, the odour of contaminated waters can be important because of the probable emission of 'rotten eggs' smells [30]; this defect is caused by the abundant presence of free sulphur amino acids.

Substantially, cheeses in water tend to spoil with increased speed compared with normal *mozzarella* cheeses. The following sensorial features should be attentively considered because of their strong connection with the real acceptability (from the viewpoint of food safety):

• Softness, gumminess, stickness
• Colourimetric modifications: from white to yellow or brown colours [30]
• Superficial defects (microblisters) by yeast fermentation
• Textural modifications
• Red pinpoint colonies on cheese surfaces by pigment producers such as *Serratia marcescens* [1]

- Excessive pH variations
- Excessive moisture values (drained cheeses)
- Unacceptable increase of the microbial spreading
- Detection of pathogen agents
- Detection of microbial toxins
- Packaging failures.

2.4 Predictive Models for Shelf Life of Cheeses

Basically, the preventive estimation of durability is mandatory from the legal viewpoint [8, 13], and the food producer or packer is entirely responsible for the correct determination of this important value. However, the evaluation of food durability values depends on various factors, including packaging materials; consequently, the HACCP approach is surely needed.

From a general viewpoint, the preventive estimation of remaining shelf life (RSL) for food and beverage products was initially carried out with the predictive microbiology. However, this peculiar approach tends to examine systematically the probable behaviour of specific spoilage life forms and the temporal advance of related processes in edible products [31]. On the other hand, the prediction of RSL should include the problem of the microbial ecology in food systems and the evaluation of peculiar chemical and physical indicators [32]. Consequently, many techniques can be used including electronic temperature integrators, data loggers and dedicated databases.

The weight of the predictive microbiology on the prediction of RSL has been predominant [31]: different mathematical models have been created and developed with the aim of describing and predicting microbial growth curves [33]. On these bases, different software products have been also created for predicting the durability of peculiar foods. Several of these programs use microbial models and chemical information at the same time.

Two examples are the Seafood Spoilage and Safety Predictor (SSSP) with reference to seafood products [34, 35] and the more general Pathogen Modeling Program (PMP). Actually, the validation of obtained predictions in 'true' conditions should be always recommended because mathematical elaborations may be related to in vitro experiments.

On the other side, RSL may be estimated by means of mathematical equations with 'chemical' inspiration like the Arrhenius law [13, 36].

In the specific cheese sector, many applications have been published. Several of these approaches are based on empiric equations: these expressions may calculate SL values of whole or portioned cheeses (different packaging materials) on the basis of chemical, physical and microbiological data [1, 2, 37].

The creation of artificial neural networks (ANN) has made possible the creation of peculiar algorithms for the prediction of SL values of processed cheeses [38]. Once more, different inputs have to be processed: yeast and mould (YM) count, pH, total viable count, soluble nitrogen content, sensory evaluations…

The prediction of SL appears correlated to many factors. This reflection may highlight the role of sensorial evaluations: the correlation between organoleptic data and the initial amount or several chemical (or microbiological) variables may be useful. In other words, the aim should be the possible creation [8] of a coherent and reliable system for the estimation of RSL on the basis of a collection of apparently disconnected variables (microbial counts, chemical compounds, sensorial scores, etc.). This approach has to discriminate received inputs: probably, much of the available information may be irrelevant, misleading or simply redundant [1]. Moreover, processing and storage conditions have to be examined: the simple record of storage temperatures can determine the validity of analytical results in terms of food hygiene [39].

Section 2.5 is dedicated to the practical application of a peculiar predictive approach. This empiric method may 'design' the SL of *pasta filata* cheeses on the basis of a few parameters: raw materials, environmental hygiene, etc. This procedure was created for *pasta filata* products in normal conditions with the exclusion of MZR in water. However, similar methods may be corrected when different products, processing and/or storage conditions are applied. Should this possibility be verified, the original approach could furnish reliable results even with relation to highly perishable cheeses.

2.5 A Peculiar Approach: Cheeses in Water

With reference to cheeses, the empiric approach to the prediction of RSL can also be used for different goals. Generally, food technologists would be able to modify cheese performances—including RSL—on the basis of the original formulation. However, several cheesemakers prefer to modify a small number of 'main' parameters (curd, salt, rennet) without the addition or subtraction of 'secondary' additives (lactic acid, etc.).

This section is dedicated to the prediction of RSL for MZR in water by means of a predictive formula for packaged *pasta filata* cheeses [1]. The related approach has been included in a free software: the 'Deductive Evaluation of Shelf-Life: Cheeses' 1.0 (DESC 1.0). Obtained results are reliable on condition that following conditions are verified [9]:

- The 'moisture on free fat basis' (MFFB) index of packed soft cheeses is >70 %.
- Packed semi-hard cheeses have MFFB ≥63 %.
- Anyway, cheeses are stored at 2 ± 2 °C (a second version of the method allows 10 ± 2 °C).

Otherwise, obtained results have to be validated [1, 2]. Moreover, following products should not be considered [9]:

- Cheeses in water
- Other cheeses under peculiar conditions: sliced cheeses, products packaged under modified atmosphere, smoked cheeses, etc.

With reference to DESC 1.0, the predictive equation is [1]:

$$[SL]_{2°C} = -1.6 \times MFFB + 29.9 \times pH - 10.9 \times \log_{10} YM \qquad (2.1)$$

where $[SL]_{2°C}$ = shelf life at 2 ± 2 °C and $\log_{10}YM$ = decimal logarithm of YM count. Actually, DESC 1.0 may use other similar equations:

$$[SL]_{10°C} = -0.7 \times MFFB + 11.6 \times pH - 2.6 \times \log_{10} YM \qquad (2.2)$$

$$[SL]_{FR} = \frac{1}{3} \times [SL]_{2°C} + \frac{2}{3} \times [SL]_{10°C} \qquad (2.3)$$

where $[SL]_{10°C}$ = shelf life at 10 ± 2 °C and $[SL]_{FR}$ means the value of RSL according to the french AFNOR V01-003 norm. The aim of this study is to calculate the food durability at 2 ± 2 °C by means of the Eq. 2.1.

As above declared, the predictive approach has been specifically elaborated for *pasta filata* cheeses but *mozzarella* cherries in water are not considered [1]. However, the chemical composition and the technology of these products are substantially identical. As a consequence, authors have decided to test the performance of the Eq. 2.1 for *mozzarella* cherries in water.

The study has been carried out near a cheesemaking industry: different productions of MZR in water have been sampled. Basically, MZR have been subdivided into two distinct typologies:

(a) A first group, named MZR-100: net weight, 100 g; gross weight, 180 g; weight of water: 80 g
(b) A second group, named MZR-250: net weight, 250 g; gross weight, 500 g; weight of water: 250 g.

All described cheeses have been produced by means of the normal 'stretching method' for MZR in hot water [18]; the final packaging has been realised with the addition of simple pasteurised water. Subsequently, produced cheeses have been sampled in the following way:

• MZR-100: five different lots, five samples per lot.
• MZR-250: five different lots, five samples per lot.

As a result, 10 different production lots have been sampled: 50 cheeses have been considered for the study and stored at 2 ± 2 °C. Chemical and microbiological analyses have been carried out in the following way.

First of all, 10 stored samples (temperature: 2 ± 2 °C) have been analysed: five lots per MZR-100 and five lots per MZR-250 cheeses, storage time: 24 h after the production date. Following analyses have been carried out:

• Moisture content (MC) of drained cheeses according to an internally validated thermogravimetric method [40].
• Fat content (FC) of drained cheeses according to the AFNOR NF V04-287 norm.
• pH value of drained cheeses with a calibrated pH-meter.

- YM count of drained cheeses according to the ISO 21527-1:2008 norm.
- Total coliform (TC) count of drained cheeses according to the AOAC 991.14 protocol.

The remaining MZR-100 and MZR-250 samples (40 total products, 20 cheeses per group, four products per lot) have been subdivided into four different groups containing one cheese per lot. The first group has been considered for analytical controls 7 days after the production date; other groups have been considered after 14, 21 and 28 days, respectively. This time, the following data have been obtained:

- pH value
- TC count of drained cheeses.

With reference to the positive or negative evaluation of cheeses in this preliminary study, acceptable products cannot show deviations from the below mentioned list of parameters:

1. Absence of unpleasant odours.
2. Absence of unusual colours.
3. Anomalous texture for the drained cheese. The product should be able to sustain the pressure of one packaged product (same weight) without ruptures for 60 s; subsequently, the cheese should return to the original shape.
4. Absence of blisters, holes, ruptures, other similar defects.
5. Absence of gaseous fermentation into the bag with consequent dilatation.
6. pH values > 6.3.
7. TC counts $\geq$ 1,000 CFU/g.

Tables 2.1 and 2.2 display all obtained results for MZR-100 and MZR-250 groups, respectively (average data). Additionally, MFFB values have been added.

Table 2.1 Analytical data for MZR-100 samples

Number of days after the production	MZR-100 samples, five different lots					
	MC	FC	MFFB index	YM count	pH	TC count
1	60.2	18.7	74.0	1.1	5.87	1.2
7					6.02	1.5
14					6.12	2.0
21					6.19	2.5
28	*Please note* expired products because of following failures: blisters and anomalous odours				6.26	2.9

All displayed data are average results. MC is for moisture (g/100 g). FC is for fat content (g/100 g). MFFB is for 'moisture on free fat basis'. YM and TC are for 'yeast and mould' and 'total coliform' respectively. The estimated shelf life (SL) at 2 ± 2 °C has been 45 days. The observed SL at 2 ± 2 °C has been 21 days

Table 2.2 Analytical data for MZR-250 samples

Number of days after the production	MZR-250 samples, five different lots					
	MC	FC	MFFB index	YM count	pH	TC count
1	59.7	19.5	74.2	1.2	5.92	1.0
7					6.07	1.6
14					6.16	2.2
21					6.24	1.8
28	*Please note* expired products because of following failures: blisters, anomalous odours, textural defects, pH values > 6.3, TC counts > 1,000 CFU/g				6.32	3.3

All displayed data are average results. MC is for moisture (g/100 g). FC is for fat content (g/100 g). MFFB is for 'moisture on free fat basis'. YM and TC are for 'yeast and mould' and 'total coliform', respectively. The estimated shelf life (SL) at 2 ± 2 °C has been 46 days. The observed SL at 2 ± 2 °C has been 21 days

Two simple deductions may be inferred on the basis of Tables 2.1 and 2.2:

1. Expired MZR-100 cheeses have shown sensorial failures, but the increase in pH and TC values is interesting and should be correlated to organoleptic defects.
2. Observed blisters and anomalous odours are surely caused by mixed fermentation, but the role of coliforms—proteolytic bacteria—should be attentively evaluated: generally, unpleasant smells were associated to the presence of sulphur amino acids.

On the other side, it has to be noted that the predictive Eq. 2.1 has calculated high SL values in comparison with the real expiration date: both MZR-100 and MZR-250 cheeses can be considered expired after 21 days, while the real date cannot be inferred (between 21 and 28 days). Consequently, the best strategy is the definition of a 'minimum' and sure RSL value: 21 days.

Differences between estimated and real RSL values were expected. However, theoretical results (45 and 46 days for MZR-100 and MZR-250 cheeses, respectively) may be mathematically corrected by means of a correction factor. In fact, real RSL correspond to 46.7 and 45.7% of calculated and erroneous RSL for MZR-100 and MZR-250, respectively. In other words, the estimated RSL may be multiplied by a number between 0.457 and 0.467 (best choice: average value, 0.462) with the aim of obtaining the real value.

Moreover, the ratio between the net weight of cheeses and the related gross weight is approximately 0.5 for MZR-100 and MZR-250: this number is similar to the supposed correction factor of 0.462.

Consequently, the original Eq. 2.1 may be corrected for MZR in water on condition that a correction factor = 0.5 is used. The chemical meaning should be evident: the higher the amount of free (and bioavailable) water, the higher the expiration of cheeses in water in comparison with normal products. More research is needed, but this hypothesis could confirm the connection between RSL of cheeses in water and the original composition of products after the production. This limitation is already evident in Eq. 2.1 because of the MFFB index [1], but the presence of free water in excess tends to reduce predictable RSL values.

References

1. Parisi S (2002) Profili evolutivi dei contenuti batterici e chimico-fisici in prodotti lattiero-caseari. IndAliment 412:295–306
2. Parisi S (2003) Evoluzione chimico-fisica e microbiologica nella conservazione di prodotti lattiero—caseari. IndAliment 423:249–259
3. Codex Alimentarius Commission (1995) Codex General Standard for Food Additives, last revision 2013. Codex Alimentarius—International Food Standards. http://www.codexalimentarius.net/gsfaonline/docs/CXS_192e.pdf. Accessed 18 October 2013
4. McSweeney PLH (2007) Principal families of cheese. In: McSweeney PLH (ed) Cheese problems solved. Woodhead Publishing Limited, CRC Press LLC, Cambridge,, Boca Raton, pp 176–177
5. McSweeney PLH, Ottogalli G, Fox PF (2004) Diversity of cheese varieties: an overview. In: Fox PF, McSweeney PLH, Cogan TM, Guinee TP (eds) Cheese: chemistry, physics and microbiology Vol 2, 3rd edn. Elsevier Academic Press, Amsterdam, pp 1–22
6. Guinee TP (2007) Introduction: what are analogue cheeses? In: McSweeney PLH (Ed) Cheese problems solved. Woodhead Publishing Limited, CRC Press LLC, Cambridge, Boca Raton, pp 384–386
7. Guinee TP (2007) Introduction: what is processed cheese? In: McSweeney PLH (Ed) Cheese problems solved. Woodhead Publishing Limited, CRC Press LLC, Cambridge, Boca Raton, pp 365–367
8. Parisi S (2002) I fondamenti del calcolo della data di scadenza degli alimenti: principi ed applicazioni. IndAliment 417:905–919
9. Parisi S (2012) Food Packaging and Food Alterations: the User-oriented Approach. SmithersRapra Technology, Shawbury
10. Pisanello D (2014) Chemistry of foods: EU legal and regulatory approaches. Springer, Heidelberg
11. Parisi S, Laganà P, Gioffrè ME, Minutoli E, Delia S (2013) Problematiche Emergenti di Sicurezza Alimentare. Prodotti Etnici ed Autenticità. In: Abstracts of the XXIV Congresso Interregionale Siculo-Calabro SitI, Palermo, 21–23 June 2013. EunoEdizioni, Leonforte, p 35
12. Parisi S (2013) Food industry and packaging materials—performance-oriented guidelines for users. SmithersRapra Technology, Shawbury
13. Parisi S, Delia S, Laganà P (2004) Il calcolo della data di scadenza degli alimenti: la funzione Shelf Life e la propagazione degli errori sperimentali. IndAliment 438:735–749
14. Donnelly CW (2007) What factors should be considered when developing a HACCP plan for cheesemaking? In: McSweeney PLH (ed) Cheese problems solved. Woodhead Publishing Limited, CRC Press LLC, Cambridge, Boca Raton, pp 146–147
15. Pritchard TJ (2005) Ensuring safety and quality I: hazard analysis and critical control points and the cheesemaking process. In: Kindstedt PS (ed) American farmstead cheese. Chelsea Green Publishing, White River Jct, pp 139–151
16. Kelly AL (2007) Introduction: how may cheese be packaged? In: McSweeney PLH (Ed) Cheese problems solved. Woodhead Publishing Limited, CRC Press LLC, Cambridge, Boca Raton, pp 159–160

17. Coles R, McDowell D, Kirwan MJ (eds) (2003) Food packaging technology. Blackwell, Oxford

18. Kindstedt PS (2007) What are pasta-filata cheeses and what physicochemical changes occur during cooking/stretching? In: McSweeney PLH (Ed) Cheese problems solved. Woodhead Publishing Limited, CRC Press LLC, Cambridge, Boca Raton, pp 300–301

19. Bottazzi V (1993) Microbiologia Lattiero-casearia. Edagricole, Bologna

20. Fédération des entreprises du Commerce et de la Distribution (2009) Critères microbi-ologiques applicables à partir de 2010aux marques de distributeurs, marques premiers prix et matières premières dans leur conditionnement initial industriel. The Fédération des entre-prises du Commerce et de la Distribution, Paris

21. McSweeney PLH (2007) How are cheese varieties classified? In: McSweeney PLH (Ed) Cheese problems solved. Woodhead Publishing Limited, CRC Press LLC, Cambridge, Boca Raton, pp 181–183

22. Alichanidis E (2007) Cheeses ripened in brine. Introduction. In: McSweeney PLH (Ed) Cheese problems solved. Woodhead Publishing Limited, CRC Press LLC, Cambridge, Boca Raton, pp 330–331

23. McSweeney PLH (2007) The microbiology of cheese ripening. Introduction. In: McSweeney PLH (Ed) Cheese problems solved. Woodhead Publishing Limited, CRC Press LLC, Cambridge, Boca Raton, pp 117–118

24. Fox PF, Guinee TP, McSweeney PLH, Cogan TM (eds) (2000) Fundamentals of cheese sci-ence. Aspen, Gaithersburg

25. Beresford TP, Fitzsimons NA, Brennan NL, Cogan TM (2001) Recent advances in cheese microbiology. Int Dairy J 11:259–274. doi:10.1016/S0958-6946(01)00056-5

26. Parisi S, Delia S, Laganà P (2008) Typical Italian cheeses and polymeric coatings. Recommended guidelines for food companies. Parts I and II. Food Packag Bull 17, 7, 8:17–21

27. Parisi S, Delia S, Laganà P (2008) Typical Italian cheeses and polymeric coatings. Recommended guidelines for food companies. Parts III. Food Packag Bull 17, 10:12–15

28. Parisi S, Caruso G (2013) Il regolamento CE 2073/2005 e successivi aggiornamenti. Studio di piani di campionamento ridotti per formaggi molli altamente deperibili. Ind Aliment (in press)

29. Parisi S, Laganà P, Stilo A, Micali M, Piccione D, Delia S (2009) Il massimo assorbimento idrico nei formaggi. Tripartizione del contenuto acquoso per mole d'azoto. IndAliment 491:31–41

30. Alichanidis E (2007) What causes softening of the cheese body in white-brinedcheeses? In: McSweeney PLH (Ed) Cheese problems solved. Woodhead Publishing Limited, CRC Press LLC, Cambridge, Boca Raton, pp 338–340

31. McMeekin TA, Ross T (1996) Shelf life prediction: status and future possibilities. Int J Food Microbiol 33:65–83

32. Benedetti S, Sinelli N, Buratti S, Riva M (2005) J Dairy Sci 88:3044–3051. doi:10.3168/jds. S0022-0302(05)72985-4

33. López S, Prieto M, Dijkstra J, Dhanoa MS, France J (2004) Statistical evaluation of math-ematical models for microbial growth. Int J Food Microbiol 96:289–300. doi:10.1016/j.ijfood micro.2004.03.026

34. Dalgaard P (1995) Modelling of microbial activity and prediction of shelf life of packed fish. Int J Food Microbiol 26:305–318

35. Dalgaard P (1995) Qualitative and quantitative characterization of spoilage bacteria of packed fish. Int J Food Microbiol 26:319–334

36. Nelson KA, Labuza TP (1994) Water activity and food polymer science: Implications of state on Arrhenius and WLF models in predicting shelf life. J Food Eng 22:271–289

37. Favati F, Galgano F, Pace AM (2007) Shelf-life evaluation of portioned Provolone cheese packaged in protective atmosphere. LWT Food Sci Technol 40:480–488. doi:10.1016/j.lwt.2005.12.001

38. Goyal S, Goyal GK (2012) Heuristic machine learning feedforward algorithm for predicting shelf life of processed cheese. Int J Basic App Sci 1:458–467
39. Parisi S (2009) Intelligent Packaging for the Food Industry. In: Carter EJ (ed) Polymer electronics—a flexible technology. Smithers Rapra Technology Ltd, Shawbury
40. Parisi S, Laganà P, Delia S (2006) Curve di crescita dei miceti in diversi formaggi in atipiche condizioni di conservazione. IndAliment 458:532–538

Chapter 3
Chemical and Health Features of Cooked Cold Meats. Reduction of Salt, Fat and Some Additives and Related Effects on Technological and Sensory Aspects of Charcuterie Products

Abstract Charcuterie products are often submitted to severe judgment because of the percentage of ingredients such as salt, fat and spices. The reduction of these ingredients is feasible in certain traditional pork cold meats, but their complete removal is difficult; otherwise, the product would lose typical characteristics. This chapter concerns *mortadella* (with relation to fat reduction) and cooked hams (with concern to salt reduction). Sodium chloride has a key role in the extraction process of proteins and with relation to the texture of cooked hams. This ingredient has been frequently substituted with potassium chloride, but this molecule may affect negatively the taste. *Mortadella* is a traditional cold meat produced with large percentage of fat cuts. Nevertheless, the manufacturing of *mortadella* has been profoundly modified in the last 20 years and the fat has been reduced without negative effects on the texture and acceptance of the product. Moreover, the use of nitrite has been discussed. The complete abolition of this additive does not seem possible at present in cooked meat products. The sensorial acceptance and microbiological features are affected by the content of nitrite in the manufacturing of cooked hams or in other charcuterie products. However, a relevant reduction of added nitrite appears to be already achieved at present.

Keywords Charcuterie product · Cooked ham · Fat · *Mortadella* · Nitrite · Sodium chloride

3.1 The Reduction of Salt, Fat and Other Additives in Charcuterie Products: An Introduction

The impact of diet on healthiness is often highlighted by researchers and the World Health Organization [1]. In particular, charcuterie products are submitted to severe judgment by both medical and nutritional viewpoints because of the high percentage of some ingredient such as salt, fat and spices or additives like nitrite. Unfortunately, the reduction of these ingredients appears feasible only in some

© The Author(s) 2014
G. Barbieri et al., *The Influence of Chemistry on New Foods and Traditional Products*, Chemistry of Foods, DOI 10.1007/978-3-319-11358-6_3

traditional pork cold meats: should the complete removal be approved, final products would lose their typical features.

Many efforts have been tried to solve these problems and meet consumers' expectations [2]. Some of these approaches are considered in this review: the reduction of sodium chloride, fat and sodium nitrite. This chapter concerns two Italian typical charcuterie products: *mortadella* (the aspect of fat reduction is mainly discussed here) and cooked hams (with reference to salt reduction).

3.1.1 Reduction of Sodium Chloride

At present, the role and the association of sodium intake with hypertension and cardiovascular diseases is well known and discussed. With relation to this matter, charcuteries are among the guilty of this contribution [3].

The main source of sodium in cooked meat products is sodium chloride, also named 'salt'. The contribution of other sodium salts—ascorbate, nitrite, polyphosphates and other additives or ingredients—is negligible [4].

Several studies have been carried out with the aim of reducing the ingoing amount of salt [5]. Obtained results have shown that the complete removal is not achievable while a significant decrease may be obtained. In addition, the elimination of salt in charcuteries may notably decrease the palatability of final products.

Basically, sodium chloride is an important ingredient that accomplishes many actions in cooked meat products: it carries out the solubilisation of salt-soluble proteins. In addition, salt preserves the product from the degradative action of spoilage bacteria and can contribute to the final taste. Finally, the reduction in cooking losses can be remarkably enhanced by means of the addition of salt.

However, some of these tasks have been maybe overestimated. For instance, the extraction of salt-soluble proteins in cooked hams can occur also with low salt percentage [6] and it seems to depend mainly on 'tumbling' step parameters, while the amount of added salt may have a secondary role. With reference to the so-called 'tumbling' process [7], the effect of processing parameters is shown by means of experimental data.

A detailed and unpublished study was carried out with relation to three different tumbling processes for the production of cooked hams (Table 3.1). The first

Table 3.1 Effect of tumbling on NaCl % content in meat at the end of the process. The presumptive amount of NaCl is calculated on the basis of % brine injection	NaCl amounts (%) at the end of tumbling processes (48 h), average results with significant difference ($p < 0.05$)		
	Presumptive amount of NaCl (%)	$T1$	$T2$	$T3$
	1.2	1.37	1.67	1.59
	1.0	1.25	1.45	1.23

Table 3.2 Effect of salt on total (TP) and myofibrillar proteins (MP) extraction in exudates and meats at the end of tumbling

	TP and MP values and standard deviations (%), in various samples at the end of tumbling processes (48 h), as correlated to NaCl amounts (%)			
	TP		MP	
NaCl amount (%)	Exudates	Meat	Exudates	Meat
1.8	10.51 ± 0.03	16.02 ± 1.18	6.70 ± 0.13	8.35 ± 0.71
1.2	10.88 ± 0.61	16.42 ± 1.13	6.50 ± 0.24	7.88 ± 2.27
1.0	10.35 ± 0.56	16.86 ± 1.69	6.02 ± 0.28	6.78 ± 2.11

two tumbling procedures, named $T1$ and $T2$, have been performed with the same friction massage into horizontal tumblers. Variations have concerned rest/work ratio values. $T1$ can be also defined as '53/7': this ratio depends on rest times, approximately 53 min, and work times (7 min). On the other side, $T2$ can be named '50/10': rest and work times are 50 and 10 min, respectively.

The tumbling system is smooth and acts through friction between the thighs. The $T3$ tumbling process provides a different mechanical action: the drum rotates on its vertical axes; thighs are (a) lifted to the upper part of the drum and subsequently (b) they fall down. Consequently, a sequence of nine cycles has been provided—15 min of work time and 45 min of rest time—followed by a long rest (15 h), also named as 'maceration step'. As a result, the total duration corresponds to 48 h. The longer the work time ($T2$ tumbling protocol), the higher the salt diffusion in meat at the end of the process. With relation to salt contents, the tumbling process surely has some influence.

Nevertheless, the obtained results have not shown significant differences when speaking of the extraction of total (TP) and myofibrillar (MP) proteins. In detail, the relationship between salt amounts and the quantity of solubilised TP and MP in the tumbling phase is shown in Table 3.2.

As a result, it may be inferred that salt contents could be reduced up to 1.0–1.2 % in cooked hams with concern to the above-mentioned relationship. The technological need for salt is lower than the current and demonstrable use, according to many scientific papers; in fact, a level of 1.7 % at least is reasonably obtainable instead of 2.3–3.0 % in several cooked hams [3, 8–10].

Since sodium chloride takes a role in the extraction of proteins and in the aqueous absorption, the influence of salt on the texture, consistency and hardness of meat products should be considered. Salt is well known for the ability to link water: this feature implies a decrease in cooking losses (Fig. 3.1). This aspect of cooked hams is extremely important when speaking of whole cut cooked meats, also called cooked roasts. On the other side, salt reduction may play a negligible role in certain processed meats such as cooked sausages because of predictable weight losses.

The influence of salt on the microbial growth is more relevant in cured and seasoned meat products compared with cooked cold meats. In fact, water activity (A_w) in cooked products may fall within a small range (0.96–0.97). In addition,

Fig. 3.1 Effect of salt content on weight cooking loss in cooked hams. This technological parameter is economically relevant and it must be taken into account

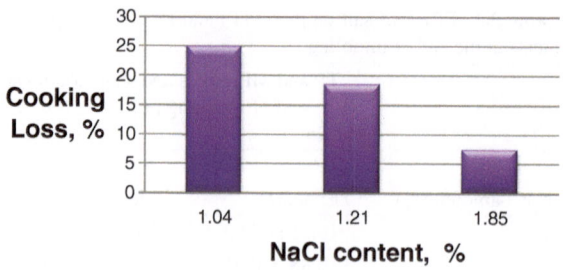

the effect of A_w on the stability of processed meat products seems low in the usual range. Consequently, these A_w values do not give any recognised microbial protection: other strategies should be tried and one of these approaches may be the substitution of sodium chloride with other substances.

A crucial aspect of the replacement of salt is the sensory acceptability of the product. With exclusive relation to cooked hams only, the organoleptic acceptance of products may decrease dramatically when salt percentages are significantly lower than a reasonable limit (1.8 %). Table 3.3 shows a selection of experimental data with concern to a sensorial test on cooked hams; this examination was performed by eight experienced panellists in the ambit of an unpublished work. The proposed score, ranging from 0 to 9, aims to represent the whole spectrum of performances, from the lower level to the higher one.

In general, sensory parameters such as brightness, greasiness, graininess, colour and compactness may be dependent on the added salt. With reference to *mortadella* sausages, it has been reported that the higher the salt content, the lower the hardness and the correlated chewiness. Similar correlations can be observed in cooked hams (Table 3.3).

Other studies have been carried out on Italian *mortadella* productions between 1990 and 2010 [11]. Generally, a significant modification of the historical and traditional formulation has been realised by means of a reduction of average salt contents from 2.56 to 2.26 % [11]. In addition, researchers have also highlighted that salt percentages were quite homogeneous in the 1990s, while the production of current *mortadella* is rather different. It may be inferred that the different approach of meat processors to food safety and health issues has progressively determined the subdivision of the original and traditional *mortadella* product in a series of versions and subversions with a broad range of salt amounts [11].

Table 3.3 Effect of salt percentage on some sensory parameters

Salt (%)	Sensory parameters, average values					
	C	CS	J	CH	S	OJ
1.8 (control)	6.35	7.52	6.57	6.35	7.45	6.55
1.2	7.40	4.50	7.00	7.15	5.50	5.73
1.0	6.35	5.12	3.85	5.65	3.15	5.33

Average values are significantly different ($p < 0.05$). *C* colour; *CS* cohesiveness of slices; *J* juiciness; *CH* chewiness; *S* saltiness; *OJ* overall judgement

Many replacements have been tested [12]. Potassium chloride (KCl) is the oldest choice; however, the complete substitution of sodium with potassium may affect negatively the taste with the concomitant and significant increase in bitterness [3]. Consequently, the partial replacement has been suggested and put into practice up to 50 % of the theoretical replacement [3]. On the other side, the assumption of high levels of potassium may affect negatively the health of diabetic patients or subjects with renal diseases. At present, KCl does not seem a conclusive solution: probably, the use of KCl can be reasonably suggested with the aim of reducing partially the sodium intake [3].

New approaches have been proposed. Hydrolysed peptides with high presence of lysine and arginine and free amino acids by the decomposition of myofibrillar and sarcoplasmic proteins can bring a salty taste in meats [13]. Alternatively, the increase in tumbling times (24–48 h) may be suggested; however, this strategy could be too expensive.

Moreover, the role of glutamic acid may be discussed. This molecule brings a peculiar *umami* savour [14] with the declared aim of misleading the taste in processed hams [15, 16]. On the other side, glutamate is involved in health concerns: for this reason the use of glutamic acid is not recommended at present.

Generally, the salty effect could be obtained by means of the presence of mineral ions and the increase of free and bioavailable water in the final product. With relation to this approach, many ingredients have been tested: phosphates, wines, some spice and ribonucleotides. A few of these ingredients are available at present; moreover, technological procedures need to be carefully revised [17].

The main factors affecting both technological aspects and sensory evaluations appear at the minimum level of sodium and fat matter. Sodium can be reduced up to a value of 1.2–1.5 % (as sodium chloride) in cooked hams with possible sensorial arrangements (flavour) and some dispensation about technological issues. On the other side, food producers have to realise and develop their own products with a certain freedom.

With concern to grounded meat products such as *frankfurter-* or *mortadella Bologna*-type sausages, the solubilisation of proteins is simpler than in whole cut muscles because the higher surface of meats can interact with ingredients. As a consequence, the diffusion of added substances is simpler and faster because of the notable addition of salt [17].

It should be emphasised that the substitution of salt in the Italian *mortadella* product is simpler than in cooked hams from the technological viewpoint: the *mortadella* processing is slightly affected by the reduction of salt. Similar to all comminuted meat products, cooking losses concern the grinding process and the fat emulsification to the same extent; on the other hand, the extraction of MP by means of the simple addition of sodium chloride (NaCl) seems less important if salt does not exceed 1.5–2.0 % [18]. Consequently, small amounts of NaCl are needed.

Mortadella-type sausages show peculiar tastes and flavours: these sensorial attributes are determined by the addition of many spices with the aim of masking easily a poor salty taste. Usually, organoleptic features of *mortadella* are 'personalised' by each food processor by means of the use of alcoholic extracts of grapes, different plants, cardamom, garlic, pepper, coriander, cinnamon, cloves, nutmeg, pimento and so on [19].

It should be also taken into account that the water content is quite low in *mortadella*-type sausages if compared with cooked hams. Moreover, the composition of lipids can notably influence tastes.

The microbiological stability of *mortadella* is achieved by means of (a) intense heating treatment and (b) adequate amount of ingoing nitrite [20]. For this reason, the reduction of salt up to 1.5–1.8 % does not appear useful: A_w decrease from 0.969 up to 0.959 with the concomitant augment of NaCl. This behaviour does not imply important improvements of the microbial stability.

3.1.2 Sodium Nitrite

The use of 'nitrite' as a food additive has been often questioned. The health toxicity of nitrites is connected to the formation of N-nitrosamine [21]; as a result, cured meat may be often considered as a health risk because of the detection of related precursors.

Nevertheless, the large number of studies focused on this issue [22] has suggested that the complete elimination of nitrite is unfeasible in cooked meat products at present [23]. Unlike seasoned sausages, cooked meat products exhibit remarkable water activity ($A_w > 0.90$): for this reason, possible pathogens could easily spread without the possibility of contrasting agents such as antagonistic bacteria.

It should be also remembered that the sensory acceptance and microbial profiles are affected by the quantitative addition of nitrite in the manufacturing of cooked hams, *mortadella* sausages and in other charcuterie products [24]. At present, the main difficulty is related to the lack of other substances with similar bacteriostatic and fat antioxidant properties. Moreover, nitrites can contribute to exhibit peculiar flavours and pink tints. However, the role of nitrites in the formation of carcinogenic N-nitrosamine and in certain reactions catalysed by iron is well known [25].

Sodium nitrite exhibits a complex chemistry because of its low stability [26]. This molecule can be oxidised and reduced following many pathways [27]. In general, three possible reactions can be considered:

$$HNO_2 + Red \rightarrow NO + OH^- + Ox \qquad (3.1)$$

$$3HNO_2 \rightarrow 2NO + NO_3^- + H_2O + H^+ \qquad (3.2)$$

$$2HNO_2 + O_2 \rightarrow 2NO_3^- + 2H^+ \qquad (3.3)$$

Basically, nitrite ion can be reduced at the lowest oxidation level. This transformation may happen in two different ways:

(a) Simple reduction to nitric oxide (reaction 3.1)
(b) Inner oxidation–reduction or dismutation (reaction 3.2) with the production of nitric oxide (NO) and nitrate.

With reference to the first pathway (reaction 3.1), the nitrite ion is initially reduced to the intermediate dinitrogen trioxide (N_2O_3). The second step is the final reduction to nitric oxide. Reducing compounds are available in meats—cysteine, glutathione, nicotinamide-adenine dinucleotide (NADH)—and others molecules (e.g. ascorbate) are usually added. As a consequence, the behaviour of nitrites is strictly connected to the redox potential and pH values in meat systems.

Another possible and non-enzymatic pathway is dismutation (reaction 3.2) of nitrous acid (HNO_2) to nitric acid (HNO_3) and nitric oxide at acidic pH values [28, 29].

A simple oxidation (reaction 3.3) needs the availability of oxygen. This reaction is not easily expected in whole meat cuts. On the other hand, oxidative processes could run to some extent in comminuted meats.

From the hygienic viewpoint, the main problem is the necessity of lowering residuals of the above-mentioned reactions: nitrites, nitrates and NO. Nitric oxide is reported to disappear just after formation [30] because of the high reactivity. Moreover, nitrite residues are often negligible or undetectable. On the other hand, nitrate is a stable anion and is reported to concern human health [31].

Consequently, the necessity of lowering nitrate (and nitrite) residues is considered crucial when speaking of food safety and meat technology. Many studies have been carried out with this purpose [23, 32].

The comprehension of the formation and the disappearance of nitrous/nitric species by the kinetic viewpoint can be useful. A specific study has been carried out with relation to nitrite and nitrate contents in cooked hams through the cooking process [33]. Figures 3.2 and 3.3 show the correlation between detected amounts of chemical anions and cooking temperatures.

Figure 3.2 concerns the influence of cooking temperatures for production of cooked hams on the amount of detected nitrate residues. With reference to this study, the maximum amount of nitrate is detected at 55 °C [33]. As regards nitrite, Fig. 3.3 displays the same type of correlation between thermal conditions and chemical levels. Once more, nitrite appears to reach maximum values when the cooking process is performed at 55 °C. However, it should be also noted that the observable decrease in nitrite residues in cooked hams throughout heat treatment does not appear linear, while the increase of nitrates (NO_3^-) in the same

Fig. 3.2 Trend of nitrate in cooked hams throughout the heat treatment process [33]

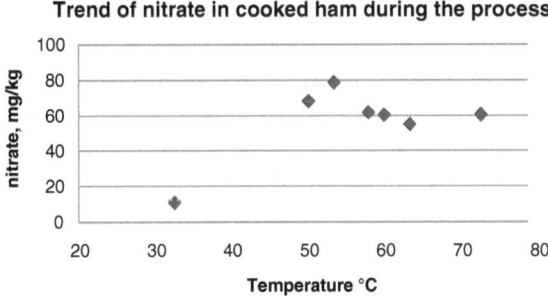

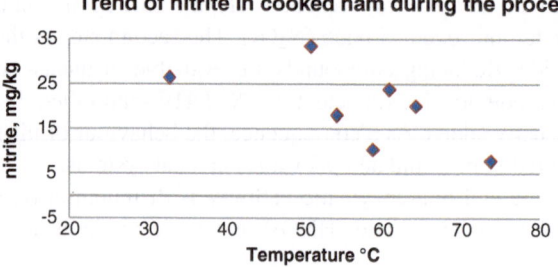

Fig. 3.3 Trend of nitrite in cooked ham throughout the heat treatment process [33]

experiment seems observable between 35 and 55 °C. After the maximum values, NO_3^- residues seem to decrease slightly [33].

The kinetics of reactions 3.1 and 3.2 has been recently studied in a real meat system, *mortadella Bologna*-type sausages, throughout the cooking process [34]. Generally, these reactions follow a first-order kinetics. As recently reported, first-order rate constants range between $1.2 \times 10^{-3} \ s^{-1}$ at 60 °C and $1.37 \times 10^{-2} \ s^{-1}$ at 70 °C for the reaction 3.1 [34]. With relation to the second reaction (dismutation of nitrous acid to nitric acid and nitric oxide), first-order rate constants have been reported between $0.8 \times 10^{-3} \ s^{-1}$ at 60 °C and $1.5 \times 10^{-3} \ s^{-1}$ at 70 °C. However, dismutation has also shown higher rate constant values at 55 °C [34].

Differently from dismutation, the reduction in nitrites is temperature-sensitive. Environmental parameters and chemical conditions, pH and redox potential values above all, become important when nitrites are detectable in many reactions at the same time.

The above-mentioned parameters can address the observable behaviour of nitrites and many other molecules in meat products. In particular, four chemical species are mainly involved, excluding nitrite:

(a) Ferric-Fe(III) and ferrous-Fe(II) ions. The associated ratio can be expressed as 'Fe(III)/Fe(II)'
(b) The ascorbate ion (HAsc⁻) and dehydroascorbic acid (DHAsc, the oxidised form of ascorbic acid). These substances are derived from ascorbic acid. This ratio can be defined as [HAsc⁻]/[DHAsc].

The evolution of the chemical system is determined by the oxidation–reduction potential (E) of every couple of involved species. It has to be considered that the influence of the concentration of hydrogen is critical for both reduction and oxidation reactions. Correlated Nerst equations are expressed as follows:

$$E = E^O - \frac{0.059}{n}\text{pH} + \frac{0.059}{n}\log\frac{[HNO_2]}{NO} \tag{3.4}$$

$$E = E^O - \frac{0.059}{n}\text{pH} + \frac{0.059}{n}\log\frac{[HNO_3]}{[HNO_2]} \tag{3.5}$$

where standard oxidation–reduction potential (E^0) values are 1.00 and 0.94 V in Eqs. 3.4 and 3.5, respectively. In addition, 'n' is for the number of electrons involved in redox reactions, namely 1 and 2 for Eqs. 3.4 and 3.5, respectively.

Basically, Eqs. 3.4 and 3.5 demonstrate that:

- Oxidised forms prevail, nitrates above all, if pH values are low.
- On the other hand, the increase in pH values determines the diminution of E and the consequent augment of reductive species, NO above all.

In addition, the slope for the E^0-pH curve is higher for the equilibrium $[HNO_2]/[NO]$ than for $[HNO_3]/[HNO_2]$.

With relation to the negative logarithm of dissociation constants (pKa), HNO_2 is reported to have a pKa of 3.40 [35]. With reference to the dissociation of nitrous acid, it may be inferred that the dissociated form, NO_2^-, is predominant when pH $\approx$ 5.75. This value is normally observed in meats. Should this pH be observed, the amount of the undissociated and reactive form—HNO_2—would be low. In fact, the ratio $[NO_2^-]/[HNO_2]$ is 2.53×10^2 at pH $= 5.75$.

The role of ascorbate ions should be highlighted. In fact, the action of nitrite depends also on the reduction to NO because of the presence of $HAsc^-$. With concern to ascorbic acid (H_2Asc), pKA is reported to be 4.17 [36]. The ratio $[HAsc^-]/[H_2Asc]$ is 3.80 at pH $= 5.75$.

In this situation, the active form is $HAsc^-$ and the meat environment allows the contemporary presence of both anionic and undissociated species. Moreover, a simple relation between the DHAsc/$HAsc^-$ redox couple and the redox potential for the correlated dissociation of DHAsc may be written as follows:

$$\log \frac{[DHAsc]}{[HAsc^-]} = \frac{E + 0.059}{0.029} \tag{3.6}$$

Equation 3.6 can be obtained from the usual Nernst equation for the DHAsc/$HAsc^-$ redox couple taking into account the pH (of meats), the number of involved electrons ($n = 2$) and E^0.

On these bases, it can be demonstrated that the predominance of reduced forms should be obtained on condition that E is lower than -60 mV. Measured E values often match similar values when speaking of meat mixtures on condition that pH is approximately 5.75. Should this value exceed 5.75, the above-mentioned predominance would be obtained with lower E (-70 mV). This deduction can be important: in fact, the equilibrium of chemical species is notably influenced by the critical pH value (5.75) above all [34]. In addition, meats may be considered as a 'strong buffering system' both for pH and E values because of the presence of one or more of these substances: glutathione, cysteine, nicotinamide-adenine dinucleotide phosphate (NADPH), etc.

It has been reported that the rate of dismutation is higher than the reduction of nitrite ions when the temperature is lower than 60 °C [34]. On the other hand, the reduction of nitrites becomes faster when temperatures go over 65 °C. With reference to the intermediate thermal range between 65 and 70 °C, nitrites appear to turn mostly into NO, while the developing nitrate ion is reduced at the same time [34].

Nitrites can be involved in different reactions with some connection to food safety and hygiene. For instance, they can react with the ascorbate anion with the enhancement of antioxidant properties [37]. Moreover, the production of N-nitrosamines can imply the presence of nitrites. Finally, the oxidative rancidity of fatty chains may be influenced by nitrites [38].

Based on the previous research, some suggestion may be inferred with reference to cooking processes: the basic aim would be the reduction of residual nitrite and nitrate particles in cold cooked meats. In detail, thermal values may be increased over 60 °C if desired results are (a) the minimisation of nitrate amounts and (b) the improvement of NO formation. It should be considered also that NO_3^- is continually generated and stable. The opposite solution—long thermal processes at low temperatures—do not seem to be helpful.

The second point of interest may concern the concentration of reducing agents, mainly the ascorbate ion, with the purpose of maintaining E values as low as possible.

At present, the current threshold limit for nitrite is 150 mg/kg in the European Union for cooked meat products that have not been sterilised [26]. However, trials have shown that the level of nitrite could be reduced at least in comminuted meat sausages. Figure 3.4 shows a peculiar product with low nitrite levels (25 mg/kg). When used for colour developing purposes, nitrite should not exceed 25 mg/kg: similar amounts are considered sufficient in cured meats to ensure the formation of nitric oxide myoglobin [39]. On the contrary, abnormal colorimetric distributions seem to be obtained with the same amount in whole cuts (Fig. 3.5).

The microbial stability of treated meats depends on the initial count of living microorganisms. At present, the European Authority on Food Safety (EFSA) has

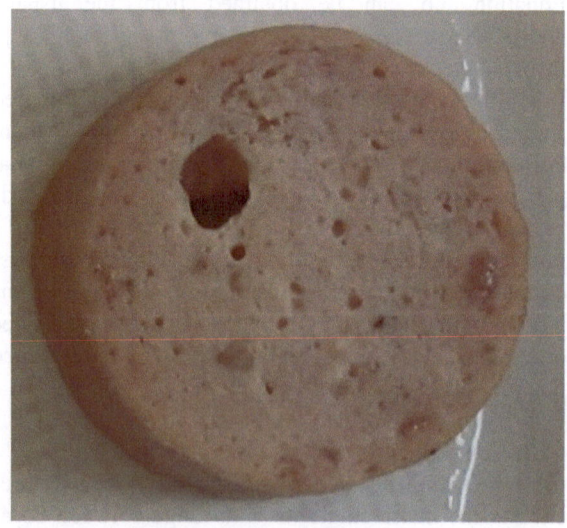

Fig. 3.4 The use of nitrite for colour developing purposes in comminuted meat sausages. A low nitrite level (25 mg/kg) can provide acceptable colorimetric results

Fig. 3.5 The use of nitrite for colour developing purposes in a whole cut (loin). Differently from comminuted meat sausages, irregular colorimetric distributions seem to be obtained with low nitrite levels (25 mg/kg) in whole cuts (Fig. 3.4)

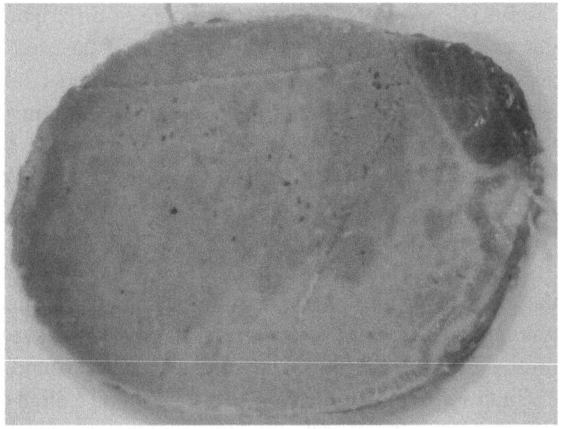

suggested a minimum ingoing amount of 50 mg/kg [40]. However, this limit may be exceeded in certain products [41].

3.1.3 Fat

Lipids are an important part of the human diet, providing a concentrated source of bioavailable energy and important compounds for the construction of cell membranes, hormones, prostaglandins and other molecules. Saturated fats can be synthesised in the human body; therefore, these compounds are not essential parts of the diet. Some unsaturated fats are considered 'essential' because they are required for specific functions and the human body cannot synthesise them. Anyway, both saturated and unsaturated fats have important functions and should be part of a healthy diet [42].

At present, a diet with approximately 30 % of the daily energy coming from the consumption of lipids is considered consistent with good human health [43]. Moreover, the amount of kilocalories from saturated fat should be reasonably low with a tolerable upper limit of 10–11 % of the total quantity of daily kilocalories [43].

People suffering from cardiovascular diseases or subject to overweight should pay attention to the consumption of fatty foods. Animal fats are often questioned because of their high content of saturated and *trans*-fatty acids. In addition, the matter of cholesterol should be considered. Modern breeding styles for pigs aim to modify the composition of animal fats. Fat reduction is a current issue to deal with.

On the other hand, the observed reduction of fat amounts in whole and comminuted meat products is quite different, depending on the formulation or used raw materials. For instance, the reduction in fat contents may be realised with the careful selection of pigs and the choice of different rearing methods when speaking of cooked hams. This strategy cannot be used for *mortadella* sausages: the decision has to be taken by the manufacturing company with regard to the possibility (and the economic convenience) of mixing cuts with less or more lean muscles.

The current decrease of fat matter in cooked hams is a consequence of new rearing protocols. Breeders would produce pigs with thin external fat layers and without exceeding 'marbling' [44–46].

In addition, leaner products can be achieved removing manually the excess of the outer fat behind the skin and the inner fat around the bone. At present, many typologies of defatted hams are on the market. Nevertheless, cooked ham is a lean product and the current fat percentage ranges around 4 %.

Tables 3.4 and 3.5 display several data on Italian cooked hams in 2010 (unpublished data). In general, low fat contents in raw meats are further reduced in cooked products after 'cleaning' processes on pig thighs. Moreover, the higher the desired quality of the final product, the higher the fat content. Normally, 'top quality' hams can be produced with the selection and the processing of heaviest thighs: main reasons are correlated to (a) the reduced thickness of superficial fat layers and (b) the upper intramuscular fat infiltration.

A further technological reduction of fat amounts can be achieved by means of the addition of starch and hydrocolloids. In fact, these molecules or compounds are known for their notable water absorption. Consequently, the addition of similar water-linking agents allows the increase of the moisture and the concomitant diminution of fat amounts in final meat products.

On the other hand, the substitution of fat matter with water can affect the physical stability of meat products: sometimes, defective meats may lose a certain amount of moisture with the consequent migration of aqueous solutions from meats to the inner surface of packages. Moreover, the insertion of water-absorbent substances among muscle fibres may be correlated with the unnatural appearance of certain ham slices because of the difference in light scattering of meat surfaces.

Table 3.4 Fat content in high-quality cooked hams and original raw thighs

	Fat content in high-quality products and original raw materials			
Food samples	Average value (%)	Minimum value (%)	Maximum value (%)	Standard deviation (%)
Raw thighs	5.39	3.56	7.25	1.29
Cooked ham	4.59	2.71	5.77	0.87

Table 3.5 Fat content in low-quality cooked hams and original raw thighs

	Fat content in low-quality products and original raw materials			
Food samples	Average value (%)	Minimum value (%)	Maximum value (%)	Standard deviation (%)
Raw thighs	4.92	4.05	5.92	0.75
Cooked ham	3.77	3.01	4.33	0.49

It has to be considered that this result may determine negative sensory evaluations by consumers, despite other situations that may occur with different causes [47].

Another point concerns the improvement of the lipidic composition by means of different feeds for pigs: the immediate modification should concern the increase of polyunsaturated fat acids. However, this option should be carefully evaluated: the diminution of the lipidic fraction known as 'low-melting fat' may be excessive. A possible consequence is the 'dripping' failure (emersion of fats and gels from the surface of treated foods and consequent accumulation) during the heating process or after packaging, in the final product.

When speaking of reduction of fat matter, more options are available in comminuted meat products such as *mortadella* or cooked sausages. *Mortadella* is an Italian traditional cold meat produced with large percentage of fat cuts. Nevertheless, the manufacture of *mortadella* sausages has evolved in the last 20 years: the reduction of fat matters in these products is reported to be higher than 10 % without negative effects for the texture and the consumers' acceptance [48].

One of the recent surveys on fat reduction demonstrated that lipids range between 19.17 and 21.94 % (unpublished results). In addition, it should be considered that *mortadella* sausages are normally produced with the peculiar insertion of little fat cubes, namely '*lardelli*', in the product. The composition of *mortadella* products should be also considered with the exclusion of *lardelli* cubes. As a result, a study has been carried out with relation to two typologies of *mortadella* sausages on the basis of the fat content (12.44 and 24.99 %). With relation to this study, a sensory evaluation has been carried out: average scores of significant attributes are shown in Table 3.6.

The diminution of fat matter seems to have a positive effect on many organoleptic aspects: taste, colour and brightness, in particular (Table 3.6). Moreover, the general acceptance seems to increase when fat is reduced (12 %). It has also been observed that sausages with high fat contents show higher salt/water ratios. In other terms, the amount of dissolved NaCl in water seems to depend strictly on the amount of fat matter with possible consequences for the consumers' perception of salty tastes.

Fat content can also affect the chromatic perception of products with a peculiar 'dilution effect': this failure is often identified with a paler pink colour of

Table 3.6 Significant differences in some sensorial parameters for two typologies of *mortadella* sausages (high and low fat levels)

Sensory parameter	High fat percentage (24.99 % on lean mixture)	Low fat percentage (12.44 % on meat mixture)	Significant difference
Graininess	7.38	7.92	$p < 0.05$
Greasiness	5.75	7.69	$p < 0.05$
Brightness	6.92	7.83	$p < 0.01$
Colour	5.88	6.69	$p < 0.01$
Taste	5.51	6.98	$p < 0.01$
Vote	5.92	6.94	$p < 0.05$

Score from 0 to 9 as hedonic evaluation

examined samples. In addition, the taste of leaner sausages has been more appreciated and slices have been judged more brilliant than usual. Probably, the last evaluation should be determined by the increasing moisture on the surface.

From the technological point of view, the quality and the chemical composition of the organic (fat) phase in meat products can become very important. In detail, a minimum value for fat matter should fall within a short range (around 10–12 %) when speaking of non-'low fat' meat systems [49]. Otherwise, meat mixtures may easily become too firm. Consequently, possible technological defects may occur in the 'stuffing' process [50]. Intermediate foods have to be forced under pressure into artificial sausage casings made from cellulose hydrate or similar materials. Should intermediate meats be firmer than usual, final products could be defective. Moreover, the heating treatment may cause some burns on the surface in the subsequent drying step: as a result, the final meat could be harder than expected.

With regard to low-fat sausages or similar processed foods, technological problems may be avoided by means of the simple augment of moisture. However, the addition of emulsifiers should be needed because final products may appear unstable. Different cooked sausages are processed with fat replacers such as hydrocolloids (xanthan, carrageenan or starch). The main role of fat replacers is to stabilise excess water in the meat system. Should this strategy be used, final meat products would be called 'light' foods. It should be noted that these ingredients are not allowed in peculiar products that are linked to a geographical area such as 'Protected Geographical Indication' (PGI) *mortadella Bologna* [51].

Other compounds have recently been suggested: vegetable fibres such as inulin and β-glucan [52, 53], canola oil [54], grape seed oil and rice bran fibres [55]. These functional ingredients may be economically convenient if the declared aim is the production of innovative cooked cold meat products. The exclusion of similar substances is definite when speaking of traditional meat products because of severe restrictions and rules, in accordance with the Regulation (EC) No 2081/1992. The above-mentioned PGI *mortadella Bologna* is one of the most known examples. Generally, a small modification of mixed cuts is allowed in these situations.

With regard to the chemical composition of PGI *mortadella* products, the following limits are compulsory [56]: the fat/protein ratio—this number has to be lower than 2.00—and the minimum amount of protein content (13.5 %). Food manufacturers are allowed to obtain a reasonable fat reduction by means of the increase of lean cuts (shoulder or lean trimmings) or other systems. However, the risk of gel accumulations has to be taken into account: in fact, the quantitative increase in connective tissues (collagenous proteins) can determine possible 'dripping' failures.

3.2 Conclusions

The content of salt, fat and nitrite in charcuterie products can be correlated with many safety aspects. The reduction of these components has been recently proposed and implemented with different results.

On one hand, fatty compounds are essential components of the original meat. In addition, NaCl can be surely considered as a traditional ingredient and preservative in many foods, including charcuterie products. On the other hand, nitrite has been questioned in recent years: many studies have been carried out with the declared aim of replacing or limiting the use of this additive in processed meats at least. However, the complete substitution of nitrite in cooked meat products does not seem to be achievable at present.

With regard to cooked meat products, the whole sequence of processing steps has to be carefully examined and regularly evaluated, step by step, because of the number of possible (desired or undesired) chemical modifications. In fact, each chemical variation of the composition and/or the physical structure of products can potentially modify the appearance and the sensory perception of the product, especially with relation to traditional (historical) cold meat products. Certainly, food consumers are able to perceive sensory characteristics of foods; in addition, they may refuse 'strange' modifications when obtained with modern technologies and ingredients.

From the industrial viewpoint, food technologists have to decide the 'right' strategy with the aim of reaching a possible agreement between economic needs of food manufacturers and sensory expectations of normal consumers: the influence of salt, fat and nitrite can affect basic organoleptic qualities of cooked meats in a predictable way.

It has been observed that cooking processes including a slow rate of increasing temperature (above 60 °C) can be useful to reduce the production of nitrate anions. At the same time, the hydrolysis of proteins is notably enhanced, improving a peculiar taste and making easier the reduction of salt.

At present, the level of salt in cooked meat products can be easily reduced by means of modification of technological processes (tumbling, cooking) and addition of suitable and allowed flavours. Many food companies are trying to turn these variations into economically convenient management strategies. From the sensory viewpoint, the contribution of nitrite and fatty compounds is not negligible.

Texture properties appear indirectly affected by the amount of salt because of the role of water as solvent. Moreover, fat content is reported to influence the hardness of meat products, especially with relation to comminuted foods. Fat matter may be often replaced with gelling agents or water-absorbing molecules such as starch or similar compounds.

The chromatic appearance is a needful property of charcuteries and the presence of nitrite ions is essential for good colorimetric results. However, the current amount of added nitrite may be notably lowered. In addition, the minimum quantity of nitrite is correlated with the microbial ecology of cooked products. Further research is needed: however, an ingoing amount of 50–60 mg/kg should be definitely considered.

Finally, the continual research and further improvements are expected to give important results in breeding and meat technology. Cooked meat products can be considered as valid and interesting carriers of proteins, essential amino acids and important elements such as zinc and iron. As a consequence, these products can be seen as both healthy foods and tasty products.

References

1. WHO (2002) The world health report. Reducing risks, promoting healthy life. World Health Organization, Geneva. http://www.who.int/whr/2002/en/whr02_en.pdf. Accessed 11 Jul 2014
2. Weiss J, Gibis M, Schuh V, Salminen H (2010) Advances in ingredient and processing systems for meat and meat products. Meat Sci 86:196–213. doi:10.1016/j.meatsci.2010.05.008
3. Desmond E (2006) Reducing salt: a challenge for the meat industry. Meat Sci 74:188–196. doi:10.1016/j.meatsci.2006.04.014
4. Ruusunen M, Puolanne E (2005) Reducing sodium intake from meat products. Meat Sci 70:531–541. doi:10.1016/j.meatsci.2004.07.016
5. Aaslyng MD, Vestergaard C, Koch AG (2014) The effect of salt reduction on sensory quality and microbial growth in hotdog sausages, bacon, ham and salami. Meat Sci 96:47–55. doi:10.1016/j.meatsci.2013.06.004
6. Bombrun L, Gatellier P, Carlier M, Kondjoyan A (2014) The effects of low salt concentrations on the mechanism of adhesion between two pieces of pork semimem-branosus muscle following tumbling and cooking. Meat Sci 96:5–13. doi:10.1016/j.meatsci.2013.06.029
7. Maddock R (2014) Meats—beef and pork based. In: Clark S, Jung S, Lamsal B (eds) Food processing: principles and applications, 2nd edn. Wiley, Chichester
8. Ruusunen M, Simolin M, Puolanne E (2001) The effect of fat content and flavour enhancers on the perceived saltiness of cooked bologna-type sausages. J Muscle Foods 12:107–120. doi:10.1111/j.1745-4573.2001.tb00303.x
9. Ruusunen M, Tirkkonen MS, Puolanne E (2001) Saltiness of coarsely ground cooked ham with reduced salt content. Agric Food Sci Finl 10:27–32
10. Food Standards Agency (2002) McCance & Widdowson's the composition of foods, Sixth Summary edn. Royal Society of Chemistry, Cambridge
11. Barbieri G, Bergamaschi M, Barbieri G, Franceschini M (2013) Survey of the chemical, physical, and sensory characteristics of currently produced *Mortadella Bologna*. Meat Sci 94(3):336–340. doi:10.1016/j.meatsci.2013.02.007
12. Omana DA, Plastow G, Betti M (2011) Effect of different ingredients on color and oxidative characteristics of high pressure processed chicken breast meat with special emphasis on use of β-glucan as a partial salt replacer. Innov Food Sci Emerg Technol 12:244–254. doi:10.1016/j.ifset.2011.04.007
13. Toldrà F and Flores M (2007) Processed pork meat flavors. In: Hui HY (ed) Handbook of food products manufacturing: health, meat, milk, poultry, sea-food, and vegetables, vol 2. Wiley, Hoboken
14. Ninomiya K (2002) Umami: a universal taste. Food Rev Int 18(1):23–38. doi:10.1081/FRI-120003415
15. Flores M, Aristoy M, Spanier AM, Toldrá F (1997) Non-Volatile components effects on quality of "Serrano" dry-cured ham as related to processing time. J Food Sci 62(6):1235–1239. doi:10.1111/j.1365-2621.1997.tb12252.x
16. Martin L, Antequera T, Ventanas J, Benıtez-Donoso R, Córdoba JJ (2001) Free amino acids and other non-volatile compounds formed during processing of Iberian ham. Meat Sci 59(4):363–368. doi:10.1016/S0309-1740(01)00088-2
17. Feiner G (2006) Meat products handbook: practical science and technology. Woodhead Publishing Ltd, Cambridge, and CRC Press LLC, Boca Raton
18. Smith DM (2001) Functional properties of muscle proteins in processed poultry products. In: Sams AR (ed) Poultry meat processing. CRC Press, Boca Raton
19. Keeton JT (2001) Formed and emulsion products. In: Sams AR (ed) Poultry meat processing. CRC Press, Boca Raton
20. Pereira AD, Gomide LAM, Cecon PR, Fontes EAF, Fontes PR, Ramos EM, Vidigal JG (2014) Evaluation of mortadella formulated with carbon monoxide-treated porcine blood. Meat Sci 97(2):164–173. doi:10.1016/j.meatsci.2014.01.017

21. Peterson LA, Urban AM, Vu CC, Cummings ME, Brown LC, Warmka JK, Li L, Wattenberg EV, Patel Y, Stram DO, Pegg AE (2013) Role of aldehydes in the toxic and mutagenic effects of nitrosamines. Chem Res Toxicol 26(10):1464–1473. doi:10.1021/tx400196j

22. Zarringhalami S, Sahari MA, Hamidi-Esfehani Z (2009) Partial replacement of nitrite by annatto as a colour additive in sausage. Meat Sci 81:281–284. doi:10.1016/j.meatsci.2008.08.003

23. Sebranek J, Bacus J (2007) Cured meat products without direct addition of nitrate or nitrite: what are the issue? Meat Sci 77:136–147. doi:10.1016/j.meatsci.2007.03.025

24. Sindelar JJ, Cordray JC, Olson DG, Sebranek JG, Love JA (2007) Investigating quality attributes and consumer acceptance of uncured, no-nitrate/nitrite-added commercial hams, bacons, and frankfurters. J Food Sci 72(8):S551–S559. doi:10.1111/j.1750-3841.2007.00486.x

25. Jourd'heuil D, Kang D, Grisham MB (1997) Interactions between superoxide and nitric oxide: implications in DNA damage and mutagenesis. Front Biosci 2:189–196

26. Honikel KO (2007) The use and control of nitrate and nitrite for the processing of the meat products. Meat Sci 78(1–2):68–76. doi:10.1016/j.meatsci.2007.05.030

27. Fox JB Jr (1966) Chemistry of meat pigments. J Agric Food Chem 14(3):207–210. doi:10.1021/jf60145a003

28. Stöhr C, Ullrich WR (2002) Generation and possible roles of NO in plant roots and their apoplastic space. J Exp Bot 53(379):2293–2303. doi:10.1093/jxb/erf110

29. Time AEA (1965) Deamination of heterocyclic amino containing compounds. US Patent 3,170,917, 24 Sept 1962

30. Lancaster JR (1994) Simulation of the diffusion and reaction of endogenously produced nitric oxide. Proc Nat Acad Sci USA 91:8137–8141

31. Pisanello D (2014) Chemistry of foods: EU legal and regulatory approaches. SpringerBriefs in Chemistry of Foods, Springer

32. Viuda-Martos M, Fernandez-Lopez J, Sayaz-Barbera E, Sendra E, Navarro C, Pe-rez-Alvarez JA (2009) Citrus co-products as technological strategy to reduce residual nitrite content in meat products. J Food Sci 74(8):R93–R100. doi:10.1111/j.1750-3841.2009.01334.x

33. Barbieri G (2013) Evolution of nitrite and nitrate in cooked meat products and their reduction in connection with the sensorial aspect. Paper presented at the 2nd BIT's annual world congress of food science and technology, Hangzhou, 23–25 September 2013

34. Barbieri G, Bergamaschi M, Barbieri G, Franceschini M (2013) Kinetics of nitrite evaluated in a meat product. Meat Sci 93:282–286. doi:10.1016/j.meatsci.2012.09.003

35. Weerasooriya SVR, Dissanayake CB (1992) Modeling the nitrosation kinetics in simulated natural environmental conditions. Toxicol Environ Chem 36(3–4):131–137. doi:10.1080/02772249209357836

36. Chih YK, Yang MC (2013) An 2, 2′-azino-bis (3-ethylbenzthiazoline-6-sulfonic acid)-immobilized electrode for the simultaneous detection of dopamine and uric acid in the presence of ascorbic acid. Bioelectrochemistry 91:44–51. doi:10.1016/j.bioelechem.2013.01.001

37. Villaverde A, Parra V, Estévez M (2014) Oxidative and nitrosative stress induced in myofibrillar proteins by a hydroxyl-radical-generating system: impact of nitrite and ascorbate. J Agric Food Chem 62(10):2158–2164. doi:10.1021/jf405705t

38. Van Hecke T, Vossen E, Bussche JV, Raes K, Vanhaecke L, De Smet S (2014) Fat content and nitrite-curing influence the formation of oxidation products and NOC-specific DNA adducts during in vitro digestion of meat. PLoS ONE 9(6):e101122. doi:10.1371/journal.pone.0101122

39. Macdougall DB, Mottram DS, Rhodes DN (1975) Contribution of nitrite and nitrate to the colour and flavour of cured meats. J Sci Food Agric 26(11):1743–1754. doi:10.1002/jsfa.2740261117

40. EFSA (2003) Opinion of the scientific panel on biological hazards on a request from the commission related to the effects of nitrites/nitrates on the microbiological safety of meat products. EFSA J 14:1–34

41. Menard C, Heraud F, Volatier JL, Leblanc JC (2008) Assessment of dietary exposure of nitrate and nitrite in France. Food Addit Contam 25(8):971–988. doi:10.1080/02652030801946561

42. Lichtenstein AH, Appel LJ, Brands M, Carnethon M, Daniels S, Franch HA, Franklin B, Kris-Etherton P, Harris WS, Howard B, Karanja N, Lefevre M, Rudel L, Sacks F, Van Horn L, Winston M, Wylie-Rosett J (2006) Diet and lifestyle recommendations revision 2006 a scientific statement from the American Heart Association nutrition committee. Circulation 114(1):82–96. doi:10.1161/CIRCULATIONAHA.106.176158

43. EuroDiet (2001) Nutrition and diet for healthy lifestyles in Europe: science and policy implications. In: Proceedings of the European conference, Crete, Greece, 18–20 May 2000. In: Kafatos AG, Codrington CA (eds) Eurodiet report and proceedings, Special issue. Public Health Nutr 4(2A):337–436

44. Armstrong TA, Ivers DJ, Wagner JR, Anderson DB, Weldon WC, Berg EP (2004) The effect of dietary ractopamine concentration and duration of feeding on growth performance, carcass characteristics, and meat quality of finishing pigs. J Anim Sci 82(11):3245–3253

45. Buege D (1998) Variation in pork lean quality. Pork fact sheet. National Pork Board, Des Moines.   http://iowapork.org/filelibrary/Factsheets/PorkScience/q-variationinporklean04522.pdf. Accessed 17 Jul 2014

46. Faucitano L, Huff P, Teuscher F, Gariepy C, Wegner J (2005) Application of computer image analysis to measure pork marbling characteristics. Meat Sci 69(3):537–543. doi:10.1016/j.meatsci.2004.09.010

47. Parisi S (2012) Food packaging and food alterations: the user-oriented approach. Smithers Rapra Technology, Shawbury

48. Beiloune F. Bolumar T, Toepfl S, Heinz V (2014) Fat reduction and replacement by olive oil in Bologna type cooked sausage. Quality nutritional aspects. Food Nutr Sci 5(7):645–657. Article ID:44062. doi:10.4236/fns.2014.57076. Available http://file.scirp.org/Html/7-2701107_44062.htm. Accessed 17 Jul 2014

49. Kerry JF, Kerry JP (2006) Producting low-fat meat products. In: Williams C, Buttriss J (eds) Improving the fat content of foods. Woodhead Publishing, Cambridge, and CRC Press, Boca Raton

50. Reichel FH (1946) Process of forming and pretesting casings. US Patent 2,401,798, 6 Nov 1946

51. Sanchez DS (2008) Supply control and product differentiation effects of European protected designations of origin cheeses. Dissertation, Kansas State University. http://krex.k-state.edu/dspace/bitstream/handle/2097/928/DeborahSanchez2008.pdf?sequence=1. Accessed 17 Jul 2014

52. Álvarez D, Barbut S (2013) Effect of inulin, β-Glucan and their mixtures on emul-sion stability, color and textural parameters of cooked meat batters. Meat Sci 94:320–327. doi:10.1016/j.meatsci.2013.02.011

53. Tomaschunas M, Zörb R, Fischer J, Köhn E, Hinrichs J, Busch-Stockfisch M (2013) Changes in sensory properties and consumer acceptance of reduced fat pork Lyon-style and liver sausages containing inulin and citrus fiber as fat replacers. Meat Sci 95:629–640. doi:10.1016/j.meatsci.2013.06.002

54. Youssef MK, Barbut S (2009) Effects of protein level and fat/oil on emulsion stability, texture, microstructure and color of meat batters. Meat Sci 82:228–233. doi:10.1016/j.meatsci.2009.01.015

55. Choi YS, Choi JH, Jeong Han D, Youn Kim H, Lee MA, Wook Kim H, Woon Lee J, Jung Chung H, Jei Kim C (2010) Optimization of replacing pork back fat with grape seed oil and rice bran fiber for reduced-fat meat emulsion systems. Meat Sci 84:212–218. doi:10.1016/j.meatsci.2009.08.048

56. Olkiewicz M, Moch P (2008) Effect of raw material formulation on basic composition and rheological properties of a model product of mortadella type. Acta Agrophysica 11(1):159–173. http://www.old.acta-agrophysica.org/artykuly/acta_agrophysica/ActaAgr_156_2008_11_1_159.pdf. Accessed 17 Jul 2014

Chapter 4
Sweet Compounds in Foods: Sugar Alcohols

Abstract Currently, there is a significant demand for food products with alternative sweeteners. Several sugar alcohols may have great potential for use in various food formulations. For instance, xylitol and other sugar alcohols have great potential as sweet compounds, which have low glycaemic indices but also benefit oral health. Continued investigation into their applications in food products will enable us to expand our realisation of the vastly undiscovered potential of sugar alcohols as alternative sweeteners.

Keywords Food formulation · Erythritol · Isomalt · Maltitol · Sorbitol · Sugar alcohol · Xylitol

4.1 Introduction

Substances eliciting the perception of sweet flavour span those classified as sugars to various compounds chemically distinct from sugar–sugar substitutes.

Sugar is a generalised term for short-chain carbohydrates of which many are used in foods and elicit sweet tastes. Furthermore, simple sugars are termed monosaccharides and include glucose, fructose and galactose. Disaccharides are obtained when two monosaccharides are covalently bonded together via a condensation reaction; they are soluble in aqueous solution along with monosaccharides. Disaccharides include sucrose (commonly referred to as 'table sugar'), maltose and lactose. Sugars of longer chain length are referred to as oligosaccharides. Generally, these molecules are produced in plant tissues via photosynthesis from carbon dioxide and water but extents of sugar production vary across species.

Sugar substitutes are natural or synthetic substances that mimic the taste of sugar (saccharose). Although the majority of approved sugar substitutes are

G. Barbieri et al., *The Influence of Chemistry on New Foods and Traditional Products*, Chemistry of Foods, DOI 10.1007/978-3-319-11358-6_4

artificially synthesised, certain bulk natural sugar substitutes are used in foods, including xylitol and sorbitol. The catalytic hydrogenation of appropriate reducing sugars is the main production strategy if the extraction of these sugar substitutes is not recommended from fruits and vegetables because of practical and economic reasons. For instance, xylose is converted into xylitol and glucose to sorbitol.

Certain non-sugar sweeteners termed 'polyols' or 'sugar alcohols' are also known. Sugar alcohols are white, naturally occurring water-soluble solids. They are typically less sweet than sucrose but have similar bulk properties and are thus attractive for use in a spectrum of food products. This chapter focuses on some of the new findings and applications of five popular sugar alcohols in food products.

4.1.1 Xylitol

Xylitol, also intended as $(2R,3r,4S)$-pentane-1,2,3,4,5-pentol, is an achiral poly-alcohol isomer of pentane-1,2,3,4,5-pentol (Fig. 4.1). Chemically, it can be produced by means of the hydrogenation of xylose [1]. D-xylose is obtained by acid-catalysed hydrolysis of vegetable matters containing xylan: this molecule is temporarily converted into D-xylulose and finally transformed in D-xylose [1].

Xylitol is widely used as a diabetic sweetener and has sweetness roughly similar to that of sucrose [1]. Owing to its increased popularity over the recent years, the number of research papers involving xylitol has grown relatively steadily (Fig. 4.2).

Interestingly, xylitol has a unique characteristic of reducing dental caries to approximately a third with regular use [2]. Several studies using data from electron microscopy have pointed towards an effectiveness of xylitol for inducing remineralisation of the demineralised enamel [3]. In addition, chewing gum with addition of xylitol has been reported to have some positive effect with concern to the reduction of acute otitis media in day-care children [4].

This compound is found naturally in fibrous tissues of various fruits and vegetables and can be extracted from materials such as birch, berries, mushrooms, oats, strawberries and cauliflowers [1, 5]. It can be also produced by recombinant microalgae [6]: in detail, the chloroplast genome of the eukaryotic microalga *Chlamydomonas reinhardtii* has been reported to be genetically engineered to yield xylitol via introduction of a gene encoding xylose reductase from a fungal

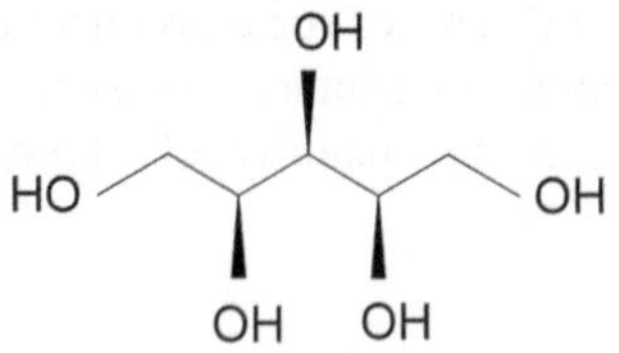

Fig. 4.1 The chemical structure of xylitol, also named $(2R,3r,4S)$-pentane-1,2,3,4,5-pentol. BKchem version 0.13.0, 2009 (http://bkchem.zirael.org/index.html) has been used for drawing this structure

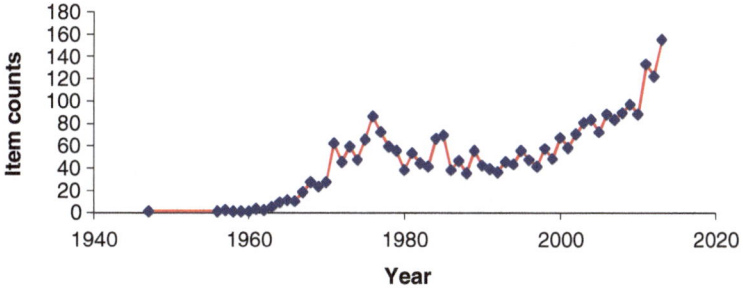

Fig. 4.2 Results counts for 'xylitol' in PubMed, 1947–2013

species. Another reported possibility is the oxidative conversion of *D*-arabitol to xylitol (intermediate product: *D*-xylulose) by means of the microbial activity of *Glucanobacter oxydans*. In detail, a dedicated *D*-arabitol dehydrogenase is used to convert initially *D*-arabitol to *D*-xylulose [7]. Subsequently, the intermediate product is turned into xylitol by means of a *D*-xylulose dehydrogenase [8]. The whole pathway does not seem to show high yields: reported values do not exceed 25 % [8, 9].

One gram of xylitol contains 2.4 kilocalories: in other words, two-thirds of the food energy for one gram of conventional sucrose [1]. Xylitol has a lower effect on blood sugar as compared with conventional sugars such as glucose: the glycemic index is reported to be 7 instead of 100 [10].

Recently, a formulation of green tea with vitamin C and xylitol has been reported to provide enhanced delivery and bioavailability of catechins in humans [11]. In detail, catechin transport measurements from both apical to basolateral and basolateral to apical directions showed an exciting potential strategy for catechin delivery enhancement [11].

Xylitol has also been shown to affect the functional properties of low-fat process cheeses [12]. Process cheese is a dairy food mixture comprised of natural cheese, salts and other ingredients heated and agitated to produce a homogenous final product. In producing low-fat cheeses, one challenge has been to overcome increased hardness and reduced melting characteristics associated with the absence of fat. Addition of xylitol has shown to significantly decrease the hardness of low-fat process cheeses as determined by texture profile analysis. Elasticity and viscosity also may improve with addition of xylitol.

4.1.2 Erythritol

Erythritol, also called (2R,3S)-butane-1,2,3,4-tetraol, is another sugar alcohol used in food products (Fig. 4.3). Like xylitol, it can be found in algae, lichens, grasses and in various fruits such as melons, grapes and pears. Erythritol is also reported

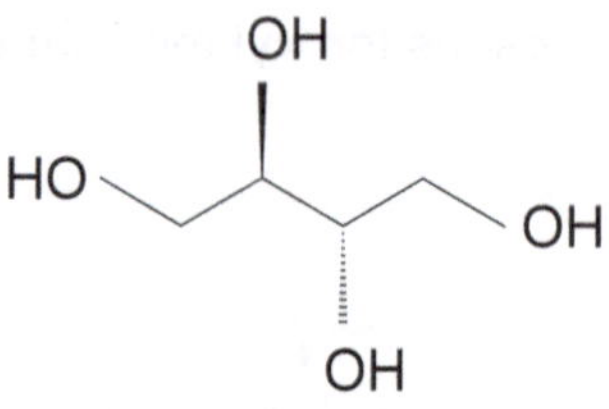

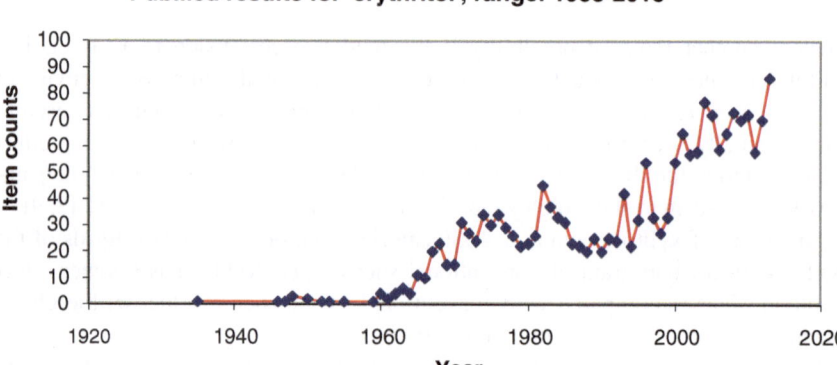

Fig. 4.3 The chemical structure of erythritol, also named (2R,3S)-butane-1,2,3,4-tetraol. BKchem version 0.13.0, 2009 (http://bkchem.zirael.org/index.html) has been used for drawing this structure

Fig. 4.4 Results counts for 'erythritol' in PubMed, 1935–2013

to be present in other foods: sake, soy sauces, etc. [1, 13]. In 2013, 87 PubMed items contained the word 'erythritol' as opposed to 156 results for 'xylitol' (Fig. 4.4).

Chemically, the structure of erythritol is peculiar because of the known achirality. Actually, the *meso*-structure shows two asymmetrical carbon atoms (2*R* and 3*S*). However, erythritol is reported to exhibit the absence of optical rotation [14]. From the viewpoint of food technologists, this molecule is well known also for the high digestive tolerance, differently from other polyols with comparable non-calorific properties [1].

Generally, erythritol is produced by means of fermentative processes. Differently from xylitol and other polyols, the hydrogenation process of carbohydrates does not seem interesting: this time, the fermentative action of fungi such as *Aureobasidium spp* or yeasts such as *Trichosporonoides spp* is preferred [1]. With relation to osmophilic yeasts, the substrate is *D*-glucose from hydrolysed starch. Resulting erythritol yields appear to be between 40 and 50 % because of the concomitant conversion of substrates to glycerol and ribitol [1].

Erythritol contains approximately 0.2 calories per gram [1]. Most dietary erythritol is absorbed into the bloodstream via the small intestine and is subsequently excreted through the urine. Approximately, 10 % enters the colon and is very unlikely to be fermented in vivo [15]. Erythritol is noncariogenic as it cannot be metabolised by oral bacteria [16]. Thus, it is a promising sugar substitute from the perspective of dental health. Recently, erythritol has been reported to have a protective effect on endothelial cells under hyperglycemic conditions [17].

Commonly, erythritol is used as a medium for delivering other sweeteners, such as stevia, to achieve a flavour similar to that of table sugar. Since erythritol is about 75–80 % as sweet as sucrose [1, 18, 19], combining it with high-intensity sweeteners can be an effective strategy for food product design. These applications are reported at present: tooth-friendly chewing gums, candy products, ice creams and also ipocaloric beverages (in association with aspartame or acesulfame K). In addition, this substance may be used as a carrier for table-top sweeteners [1, 20, 21]. Erythritol is not hygroscopic and thus does not attract moisture. This is an important characteristic to keep in mind as it may necessitate the use of other hygroscopic components in product formulations.

4.1.3 Maltitol

Maltitol, also called 4-O-α-D-glucopyranosyl-D-glucitol, is reported to have a relative sweetness of approximately 0.65, although 0.9 may be signalled [1, 22]. It contains 2.1 calories per gram: this ipocaloric value is reported to be lower if maltitol is compared with sucrose [1]. In addition, maltitol is highly stable by the thermal and chemical viewpoint and exhibits very similar properties to table sugar: viscosity (when dissolved in aqueous solutions), hygroscopicity, solubility in water, etc. [1, 23]. It is commonly produced via a hydrogenation method involving starch-obtained maltose. Furthermore, maltitol syrup is made by hydrogenation of mixed carbohydrates from starch. The high sweetness level of maltitol lends itself well to being incorporated in sweets and candy products, chocolates, ice creams, etc. [1].

Chemically, maltitol is different from the above-mentioned polyols because of the peculiar structure: this molecule is a disaccharide where a glucose heteroatomic ring is connected with a sorbitol unit [1].

Maltitol has a documented laxative effect when consumed in large quantities. However, it has been recently reported that osmotic diarrhoea caused by maltitol ingestion could be suppressed by adding soluble or insoluble fibre to ingested maltitol products [24]. More recently, the concomitant use of maltitol and short-chain fructo-oligosaccharides has been suggested in sugar-free food product formulations to lower postprandial glycaemic responses [25]. Finally, the positive action of maltitol has been demonstrated in rats with concern to the absorption of intestinal calcium [1, 26].

In spite of the interesting properties of this molecule, only 199 total results are counted for searching the key word 'maltitol' on PubMed until 2013.

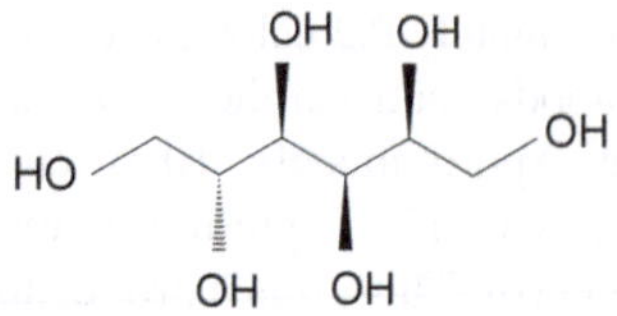

Fig. 4.5 The chemical structure of sorbitol, also named (2S,3R,4R,5R)-Hexane-1,2,3,4,5,6-hexol. BKchem version 0.13.0, 2009 (http://bkchem.zirael.org/index.html) has been used for drawing this structure

4.1.4 Sorbitol

Sorbitol or (2*S*,3*R*,4*R*,5*R*)-hexane-1,2,3,4,5,6-hexol is also known as glucitol (Fig. 4.5). After metabolisation, this alcohol can provide 2.6 calories per gram. Chemically, it can be obtained [1] by:

- Electrochemical reduction of dextrose in alkaline conditions. During the reduction of glucose, the aldehyde group is changed to a hydroxyl group. However, a notable content of mannitol is obtained also because of the observed epimerisation of dextrose to fructose.
- High-pressure catalytic hydrogenation of dextrose (mannitol does not exceed 2 %).
- Catalytic hydrogenation of sucrose (mannitol is also produced).

Sorbitol is mainly produced from corn syrup but can also be found in various fruits such as berries, peaches, apples and pears [27]. Interestingly, sorbitol plays an important role in carbon metabolism of fruits and affects the quality of starch accumulation and sugar–acid balance. Sorbitol as a key search word on PubMed draws the following result counts by year (Fig. 4.6).

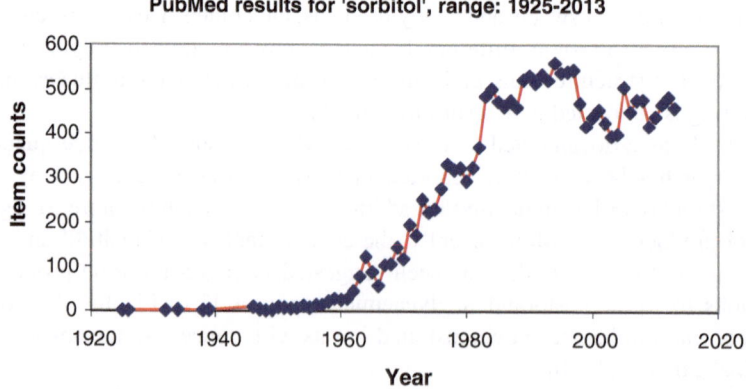

Fig. 4.6 Results counts for 'sorbitol' in PubMed, 1925–2013

Sorbitol, like other sugar alcohols such as maltitol, can have a laxative effect. In fact, the well-known laxative effect of prunes may be explained by their high sorbitol content: 14.7 g/100 g [28]. Sorbitol-based osmotic diarrhoea has been shown to be the result of intestinal malabsorption. In rats, rice starch contained in rice gruel may cause a slower rate of intestinal transit of sorbitol when ingested together [29]. Moreover, this slower gastric emptying and intestinal transit may help to maintain a constant normal osmotic environment in the intestinal lumen so as to prevent diarrhoea.

Owing to its thickening and humectant properties, sorbitol can be and is used in food (and even cosmetic) formulations which necessitate those properties. Since sorbitol has a high enough refractive index, it may be used for formulation of transparent substances. In addition, 25 % of the total production of sorbitol is reported to be destined for the realisation of syrups (moisture stabilisers and softeners) [1, 30].

4.1.5 Isomalt

Isomalt, also called (2R,3R,4R,5R)-6-[[(2S,3R,4S,5S,6R)- 3,4,5-trihydroxy-6-(hydroxymethyl)- 2-tetrahydropyranyl]oxy]hexane- 1,2,3,4,5-pentol, has 2 calories per gram and has similar physical properties as sugar. It is an equimolar mixture of two disaccharides, each composed of glucose and mannitol. Isomalt is typically manufactured by transformation of sucrose into isomaltulose which is then subsequently hydrogenated. Isomalt does not crystallise as quickly as sucrose and is thus attractive for use in sugar sculpture and other decorative edible products.

Isomalt (Fig. 4.7) appears to be a palatable alternative sweetener for use in diabetic confectionaries as it exhibits a lower glycaemic effect (0.45) in comparison to conventional chocolate [31]. In addition, isomalt is reported to give higher specific heat capacity, lower viscosity and higher boiling point values to melted preparations when added. Finally, the high stability to acid hydrolysis is well known: for these and other reasons, the use of isomalt is recommended in many food and non-food applications if compared with other polyol sweeteners [1, 32].

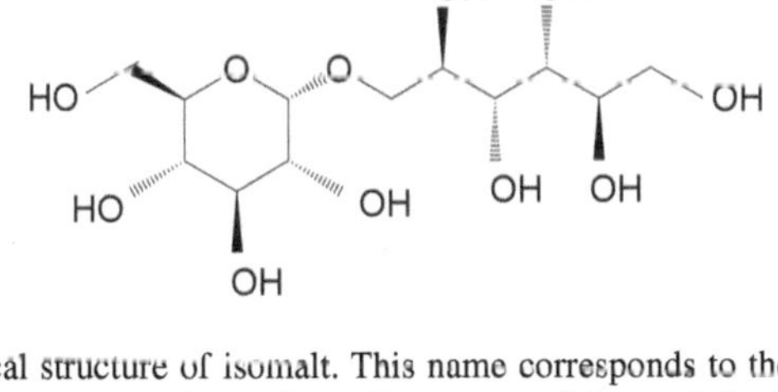

Fig. 4.7 The chemical structure of isomalt. This name corresponds to the mixture of two diastereoisomers in different proportions, depending on conditions of the hydrogenation of isomaltulose by sucrose via enzymatic reaction. BKchem version 0.13.0, 2009 (http://bkchem.zirael .org/index.html) has been used for drawing this structure

References

1. Evrendilek GA (2012) Sugar alcohols (Polyols). In: Varzakas T, Labropoulos A, Anestis S (eds) Sweeteners: nutritional aspects, applications, and production technology. CRC Press, Boca Raton
2. Steinberg LM, Odusola F, Mandel ID (1992) Remineralizing potential, antiplaque and antig-ingivitis effects of xylitol and sorbitol sweetened chewing gum. Clin Prev Dent 14(5):31–34
3. Miake Y, Saeki Y, Takahashi M, Yanagisawa T (2003) Remineralization effects of xylitol on demineralized enamel. J Electron Microsc 52(5):471–476. doi:10.1093/jmicro/52.5.471
4. Uhari M, Tapiainen T, Kontiokari T (2000) Xylitol in preventing acute otitis media. Vaccine 19(Suppl 1):144–147. doi:10.1016/S0264-410(00)00294-2
5. Johansson B, Christensson C, Hobley T, Hahn-hägerdal B (2001) Xylulokinase overexpression in two strains of Saccharomyces cerevisiae also expressing xylose reductase and xylitol dehydrogenase and its effect on fermentation of xylose and lignocellulosic hydrolysate. Appl Environ Microbiol 67(9):4249–4255. doi:10.1128/AEM.67.9.4249-4255.2001
6. Pourmir A, Noor-Mohammadi S, Johannes TW (2013) Production of xylitol by recombinant microalgae. J Biotechnol 165(3–4):178–183. doi:10.1016/j.jbiotec.2013.04.002
7. Koganti S, Kuo TM, Kurtzman CP, Smith N, Ju LK (2011) Production of arabitol from glycerol: strain screening and study of factors affecting production yield. Appl Microbiol Biotechnol 90(1):257–267. doi:10.1007/s00253-010-3015-3
8. Suzuki S, Sugiyama M, Mihara Y, Hashiguchi K, Yokozeki K (2002) Novel enzymatic method for the production of xylitol from Darabitol by Gluconobacter oxydans. Biosci Biotechnol Biochem 66(12):2614–2620. doi:10.1271/bbb.66.2614
9. Sugiyama M, Suzuki S, Tonouchi N, Yokozeki K (2003) Cloning of the xylitol dehydrogenase gene from gluconobacter oxydans and improved production of xylitol from D-arabitol. Biosci Biotechnol Biochem 67(3):584–591. doi:10.1271/bbb.67.584
10. Foster-Powell K, Holt SH, Brand-Miller JC (2002) International table of glycemic index and glycemic load values: 2002. Am J Clin Nutr 76(1):5–56
11. Chung JH, Kim S, Lee SJ, Chung JO, Oh YJ, Shim SM (2013) Green tea formulations with vitamin C and xylitol on enhanced intestinal transport of green tea catechins. J Food Sci 78(5):C685–C690. doi:10.1111/1750-3841.12112
12. Kommineni A, Amamcharla J, Metzger LE (2012) Effect of xylitol on the functional properties of low-fat process cheese. J Dairy Sci 95(11):6252–6259. doi:10.3168/jds.2012-5376
13. Robyt JF (1998) Essentials of carbohydrate chemistry. Springer, New York
14. Montero CM, Dodero MR, Sánchez DG, Barroso CG (2004) Analysis of low molecular weight carbohydrates in food and beverages: a review. Chromatographia 59(1–2):15–30. doi:10.1365/s10337-003-0134-3
15. Arrigoni E, Brouns F, Amadò R (2005) Human gut microbiota does not ferment erythritol. Br J Nutr 94(5):643–646. doi:10.1079/BJN20051546
16. Kawanabe J, Hirasawa M, Takeuchi T, Oda T, Ikeda T (1992) Noncariogenicity of erythritol as a substrate. Caries Res 26(5):358–362. doi:10.1159/000261468
17. Boesten DM, Berger A, de Cock P, Dong H, Hammock BD, den Hartog GJ, Bast A (2013) Multi-targeted mechanisms underlying the endothelial protective effects of the diabetic-safe sweetener erythritol. PLoS ONE 8(6):e65741. doi:10.1371/journal.pone.0065741
18. Ishizuka H, Wako K, Kasumi T, Sasaki T (1989) Breeding of a mutant of Aureobasidium sp. with high erythritol production. J Ferment Bioeng 68(5):310–314. doi: 10.1016/0922-338(89)90003-2
19. Jeya M, Lee KM, Tiwari MK, Kim JS, Gunasekaran P, Kim SY, Kim IW, Lee JK (2009) Isolation of a novel high erythritol-producing Pseudozyma tsukubaensis and scale-up of erythritol fermentation to industrial level. Appl Microbiol Biotechnol 83(2):225–231. doi:10.1007/s00253-009-1871-5
20. Boileau A, Fry JC, Murray R (2012) A new calorie-free sugar substitute from the leaf of the stevia plant arrives in the UK. Nutr Bull 37(1):47–50. doi:10.1111/j.1467-3010.2011.01945.x/full

21. Catani SJ, Navia JL (2012) Method of making an enhanced natural sweetener. US Patent 13,367,650 9 Aug 2012
22. Schiffman SS, Booth BJ, Losee ML, Pecore SD, Warwick ZS (1995) Bitterness of sweeteners as a function of concentration. Brain Res Bull 36(5):505–513. doi:10.1016/0361-9230(94)00225-P
23. Sokmen A, Gunes G (2006) Influence of some bulk sweeteners on rheological properties of chocolate. LWT-Food Sci Technol 39(10):1053–1058. doi:10.1016/j.lwt.2006.03.002
24. Oku T, Hongo R, Nakamura S (2008) Suppressive effect of cellulose on osmotic diarrhea caused by maltitol in healthy female subjects. J Nutr Sci Vitaminol 54(4):309–314
25. Respondek F, Hilpipre C, Chauveau P, Cazaubiel M, Gendre D, Maudet C, Wagner A (2014) Digestive tolerance and postprandial glycaemic and insulinaemic responses after consumption of dairy desserts containing maltitol and fructo-oligosaccharides in adults. Eur J Clin Nutr 68:575–580. doi:10.1038/ejcn.2014.30
26. Goda T, Takase S, Hosoya N (1993) Maltitol-induced increase of transepithelial transport of calcium in rat small intestine. J Nutr Sci Vitaminol 39(6):589–595
27. Teo G, Suzuki Y, Uratsu SL, Lampinen B, Ormonde N, Hu WK, DeJong TM, Dandekar AM (2006) Silencing leaf sorbitol synthesis alters long-distance partitioning and apple fruit quality. Proc Natl Acad Sci USA 103(49):18842–18847. doi:10.1073/pnas.0605873103
28. Stacewicz-Sapuntzakis M, Bowen PE, Hussain EA, Damayanti-wood BI, Farnsworth NR (2001) Chemical composition and potential health effects of prunes: a functional food? Crit Rev Food Sci Nutr 41(4):251–286. doi:10.1080/20014091091814
29. Islam MS, Sakaguchi E (2006) Sorbitol-based osmotic diarrhea: possible causes and mechanism of prevention investigated in rats. World J Gastroenterol 12(47):7635–7641
30. Schiweck H, Bär A, Vogel R, Schwarz E, Kunz M, Dusautois C, Clement A, Lefranc C, Lüssem B, Moser M, Peters S(1999) Sugar alcohols. Ullmann's encyclopedia of industrial chemistry. Wiley, Weinheim. doi:10.1002/14356007.a25_413.pub3
31. Gee JM, Cooke D, Gorick S, Wortley GM, Greenwood RH, Zumbé A, Johnson IT (1991) Effects of conventional sucrose-based, fructose-based and isomalt-based chocolates on postprandial metabolism in non-insulin-dependent diabetics. Eur J Clin Nutr 45(11):561–566
32. Rapp KM, Willibald-Ettle I (2005) Sugar-free pharmaceutical products. US Patent 6,872,415 29 Mar 2005

Chapter 5
Food Manufacturing and Allergen Management

Keywords Antigen · Antibody · Epitope · Allergenicit · Risk management · Cross-contamination

5.1 Introduction to Food Allergens

Allergens are naturally occurring proteins responsible for causing non-toxic immune mediated adverse food reaction, called 'Food Allergy', in consumers. Another type of non-toxic reactions is 'Food Sensitivity or Intolerance'. Allergic reactions such as anaphylactic shocks may even cause death within minutes. For these and other reasons, medical treatments are urgently required. Multiple factors are involved in development of allergies like genetics, age, dose, exposure to allergenic foods, etc. The aim of this chapter is to provide a general overview of the problem of food allergens in the current food industry with a description of main countermeasures.

From a general viewpoint, food allergy has been observed and identified as a clinical concern since 1921 [1–4]. On the other hand, hygienists have progressively considered this phenomenon as a public health problem instead of individual incidents with food-related causes in the last 30 years [5–8].

The problem of food allergy as a systematic phenomenon with non-aleatory causes can be observed and studied with different approaches. One of these methods can be simply referred to the numerical dimension or magnitude of observed situations. In other words, the following factors should be considered by a clinical viewpoint [8]:

- The prevalence of the allergic condition with a necessary connection to safety consequences on the human being, and
- Limits of responsibility for the different players or stakeholders of the so-called 'food chain'.

With regard to the first factor, it has been reported that 1–2 % of the population may suffer from food allergic reactions. In addition, the exposure may reach 8 %

© The Author(s) 2014
G. Barbieri et al., *The Influence of Chemistry on New Foods and Traditional Products*, Chemistry of Foods, DOI 10.1007/978-3-319-11358-6_5

in case of children [8–11]. On the other hand, the perceived extension of the food allergic condition may be notably underestimated [8, 12] because of:

(a) The similarity between allergic reactions within a single family [13]. As a result, the totality of the members of a single and restricted community can have a peculiar food allergy; on the other hand, only a few cases might be reported.
(b) Self-reported food allergic reactions appear to be greater than the estimated and clarified prevalence of 'official' results [14].
(c) Different people eat different foods and a variety of different branded edible products. As a consequence, the penetration of a peculiar food in the market can affect possible studies and simulations about allergy risks, depending on reasons such as the regionality of brands [15].

The problem of food allergy may be notably complicated when considering the number of possible players of the food chains and related responsibilities. With the preventive exclusion of consumers' duties, medical exceptions and the behaviour of mass retailers and distributors, the main responsibilities of food producers may be summarised as follows [8, 16]:

• The food industry must provide safe foods (general requirement) without exclusions, including the possibility of food allergy- sensitive consumers. This obligation is mainly carried out by means of adequate 'good manufacturing practices' [15] with the aim of removing known food allergens from the supply chain (if possible).
• Moreover, food producers have to inform potentially sensitive consumers with adequate labels or interactive systems. Basically, this information is compulsory in many countries and macroeconomic regions with concern to simple labelling descriptions.
• Finally, the food industry should carefully evaluate the use of novel foods or ingredients because of possible food allergic reactions. For this reason, trial tests should be carried out in the so-called 'design' step of foods before production, with the aim of preventing worst case scenarios [17]. For example, could a specified novel food cause allergic reactions and/or increase the estimated food allergy prevalence in the normal population? Because of the lack of predictive tests for the identification of potential allergenicity by novel foods (especially proteins), these 'ingredients' should be evaluated as potential allergens [8].

5.2 Chemistry and Action of Allergens

Allergy may be defined as the result of binding between 'epitopes'—peculiar regions of tridimensional proteins—and the so-called ε heavy chain- immunoglobulin (IgE) [18, 19]. Every epitope can be considered as a molecular region on the surface of an 'antigen' with the ability of causing a specific reaction or 'response' by an 'antibody' molecule. As a consequence, a specific epitope is recognized by a specific 'antibody' or antigen receptor. For these reasons, epitopes can also be called antigenic determinants because of the localization into a molecule—the antigen—with the ability of generating specific antibodies [18, 19].

As a result, allergic reactions correspond to the response of environmental antigens when in presence of pre-existing antibodies. Allergy may be observed in a variety of situations; on the other hand, the most known mechanism appears the binding of allergen epitopes to IgE antibody on mast cells. Observed consequences may be asthma, allergic rhinitis, etc., because of the occurrence of the so-called 'immediate reaction' (a few seconds are needed) [19]. However, the systematic exposure to antigens may also cause anaphylactic shocks with consequent circulatory collapses and suffocation due to tracheal swelling [19]. These reactions occur within minutes of exposure. Consequently, effects are observed with a certain delay as compared to immediate reactions.

In addition, the increased tendency to produce immediate hypersensitivity reactions against potential allergens, the so-called 'atopic' allergy, is one of the growing fields of interest [18, 19].

Chemically, the reaction between IgE normally present in human serum in extremely small quantities, although serum concentration may increase several hundred if specific stimuli are given [20–22]—and allergens is typically persistent because of the high-affinity receptor FcεRI [23] in basophils and mast cells, and the low-affinity receptor FcεRII [24]. Consequently, the presence of allergens—usually water-soluble glycoproteins with molecular weights between 10 and 70 kDalton—can determine the release of chemicals like histamines and leukotrienes with the occurrence of above-mentioned 'immediate' symptoms [24].

Food allergens may resist heat, acids and proteases. One of these examples is the Ara h 1 glycoprotein: this molecule—a highly structured protein with a clear tertiary fold and reported to be found as a trimeric complex in peanuts—is reported to exhibit excellent stability to heat, in spite of the clear denaturation by digestive enzymes [24, 25]. As a result, the allergenicity of Ara h 1 may appear unaffected by thermal treatments. In addition, related allergic reactions may occur with a dose of 100 µg with the risk of severe dangers for subjects with peanut allergy [25].

The above shown situation may be observed with other food allergens. As a clear result, the approach to allergen risk management in the food industry is expected to be mainly focussed on the implementation of good manufacturing practices, including correct guidelines for the handling of allergens and the exclusion of cross-contamination [8]. In other words, food allergenicity cannot be reasonably curtailed by processing procedures such as thermal treatments or 'enzymatic' strategies.

5.3 Food Allergens and the Industry: Risk Management

Because of lack of processes or technical solutions for the eradication of food allergenicity, the current approach appears mainly focussed on the information to consumers (labelling) and the concomitant limitation of all possible allergens in food until a safe value can be reached [8].

On the other hand, it should be recognised that:

- Mentioning a peculiar food allergen may be difficult. As a consequence, the term 'lactose' can be identified under the more general 'milk and milk products, including lactose' phrase. Thus, all possible milk derivatives would be named with the same efficacy. This is the current position in the European Union (EU) [26]
- The quantitative limitation of allergens in industrial productions and recipes can be obtained by cooperative efforts. Subsequently, the exclusion of allergenic substances should be assured by means of continuous and regular controls by suppliers and manufacturers of food products. This monitoring activity should be managed by brand-owner and non-manufacturing companies by means of detailed audits, in accordance with food safety system protocols such as ISO 22000 and other standards by British Retail Consortium and International Featured Standards (IFS). The Regulation (EU) No 1169/2011 defines the position of brand-owners with well-circumscribed responsibilities with respect to labelling declarations. As a result, the control on manufacturing should be performed by the totality of involved players
- The problem of cross-contamination is critical. The management of this risk is generally considered by means of the 'hazard analysis and critical control points' (HACCP) approach. However, HACCP plans need to be constantly reviewed with the aim of assuring that all possible risks are reduced to an acceptable level. In addition, prerequisite programmes as cleaning and sanitation & allergen control policy—are the foundation of the HACCP plans [27].

In conclusion, the management of food allergens is a work in progress. Because of the notable number of food allergen-related alerts in the EU, new strategies are needed. The necessity for repeated audits and the validation of new and cost-effective analytical protocols for different food matrices continue to be the economic challenge for allergen management [27].

References

1. Duke WW (1921) Food allergy as a cause of abdominal pain. Arch Intern Med (Chic) 28(2):151–165. doi:10.1001/archinte.1921.00100140028003
2. Rowe AH (1928) Food allergy: its manifestations, diagnosis and treatment. J Am Med Assoc 91(21):1623–1631. doi:10.1001/jama.1928.02700210037011
3. Tuft L, Blumstein GI (1942) Studies in food allergy: II. sensitization to fresh fruits: clinical and experimental observations. J Allerg 13:574–582. doi:10.1016/S0021-8707(42)90070-4
4. Loveless MH (1950) Milk allergy: a survey of its incidence; experiments with a masked ingestion test. J Allerg 21:489–499
5. Sicherer SH (2011) Epidemiology of food allergy. J Allergy Clin Immunol 127(3):594–602. doi:10.1016/j.jaci.2010.11.044
6. Boyce JA, Assa'ad A, Burks AW, Jones SM, Sampson HA, Wood RA, Plaut M, Cooper SF, Fenton MJ, Arshad SH, Bahna SL, Beck LA, Byrd-Bredbenner C, Camargo CA Jr, Eichenfield L, Furuta GT, Hanifin JM, Jones C, Kraft M, Levy BD, Lieberman P, Luccioli S, McCall KM, Schneider LC, Simon RA, Simons FE, Teach SJ, Yawn BP, Schwaninger JM (2010) Guidelines for the diagnosis and management of food allergy in the United States:

report of the NIAID-sponsored expert panel. J Allergy Clin Immunol 126(6 Suppl):S1–S58. doi:10.1016/j.jaci.2010.10.007

7. Holgate ST (1999) The epidemic of allergy and asthma. Nature 402(6760 Suppl):B2–B4
8. Crevel R (2002) Industrial dimensions of food allergy. Biochem Soc Trans 30(6):941–944
9. Bock SA, Atkins FM (1990) Patterns of food hypersensitivity during sixteen years of double-blind, placebo-controlled food challenges. J Pediatr 117(4):561–567
10. Young E, Stoneham MD, Petruckevitch A, Barton J, Rona R (1994) A population study of food intolerance. Lancet 343(8906):1127–1130. doi:10.1016/S0140-6736(94)90234-8
11. Rhodes HL, Thomas P, Sporik R, Holgate ST, Cogswell JJ (2002) A birth cohort study of subjects at risk of atopy: twenty-two-year follow-up of wheeze and atopic status. Am J Respir Crit Care Med 165:176–180. doi:10.1164/ajrccm.165.2.2104032
12. Altman DR, Chiaramonte LT (1996) Public perception of food allergy. J Allergy Clin Immunol 97(6):1247–1251. doi:10.1016/S0091-6749(96)70192-6
13. Emmett SE, Angus FJ, Fry JS, Lee PN (1999) Perceived prevalence of peanut allergy in Great Britain and its association with other atopic conditions and with peanut allergy in other household members. Allergy 54(4):380–385. doi:10.1034/j.1398-9995.1999.00768.x
14. Sicherer SH, Furlong TJ, DeSimone J, Sampson HA (1999) Self-reported allergic reactions to peanut on commercial airliners. J Allergy Clin Immunol 104(1):186–189. doi:10.1016/S0091-6749(99)70133-8
15. Parisi S (2013) Food packaging and food alterations. Smithers Rapra Technology, Shawbury
16. Houghton JR, Rowe G, Frewer LJ, Van Kleef E, Chryssochoidis G, Kehagia O, Korzen-Bohr S, Lassen J, Pfenning U, Strada A (2008) The quality of food risk management in Europe: perspectives and priorities. Food Policy 33(1):13–26. doi:10.1016/j.foodpol.2007.05.001
17. Hepburn P, Howlett J, Boeing H, Cockburn A, Constable A, Davi A, de Jong N, Moseley B, Oberdörfer R, Robertson C, Wal JM, Samuels F (2008) The application of post-market monitoring to novel foods. Food Chem Toxicol 46(1):9–33. doi:10.1016/j.fct.2007.09.008
18. Singh AB, Kumar P (2003) Aeroallergens in clinical practice of allergy in India. An Overview. Ann Agric Environ Med 10(2):131–136
19. Janeway CA Jr, Travers P, Walport M, Shlomchik MJ (2001) Immunobiology: the immune system in health and disease, 5th edn. Garland Science, New York. Glossary. http://www.ncbi.nlm.nih.gov/books/NBK10759/. Accessed 20 May 2014
20. Agha F, Sadaruddin A, Abbas S, Ali SM (1997) Serum IgE levels in patients with allergic problems and healthy subjects. J Pak Med Assoc 47(6):166–169
21. Ishizaka K, Ishizaka T, Hornbrook MM (1967) Allergen-binding activity of gamma-E, gamma-G and gamma-A antibodies in sera from atopic patients. In vitro measurements of reaginic antibody. J Immunol 98:490–492
22. Wide L, Bennich H, Johansson SGO (1967) Diagnosis of allergy by an in-vitro test for allergen antibodies. Lancet 290(7526):1105–1107. doi:10.1016/S0140-6736(67)90615-0
23. Beaven MA, Baumgartner RA (1996) Downstream signals initiated in mast cells by Fc epsilon RI and other receptors. Curr Opin Immunol 8(6):766–772
24. Cianferoni A, Spergel JM (2009) Food allergy: review, classification and diagnosis. Allergol Int 58(4):457–466. doi:10.2332/allergolint.09-RAI-0138
25. Koppelman SJ, Bruijnzeel-Koomen CA, Hessing M, de Jongh HH (1999) Heat-induced conformational changes of Ara h 1, a major peanut allergen, do not affect its allergenic properties. J Biol Chem 274(8):4770–4777
26. Wróblewska B, Jedrychowski L (2012) Milk Allergens. In: Jedrychowski L, Wichers HJ (eds) Chemical and biological properties of food allergens. CRC Press, Boca Raton
27. Kerbach S, Alldrick AJ, Crevel RW, Dömötör L, DunnGalvin A, Clare Mills EN, Pfaff S, Poms RE, Popping B, Tömösközi S (2009) Managing food allergens in the food supply chain–viewed from different stakeholder perspectives. Qual Assur Saf Crops Foods 1(1):50–60. doi:10.1111/j.1757-837X.2009.00009.x